Management of Medication-related Osteonecrosis of the Jaw

Editor

SALVATORE L. RUGGIERO

ORAL AND MAXILLOFACIAL SURGERY CLINICS OF NORTH AMERICA

www.oralmaxsurgery.theclinics.com

Consulting Editor
RICHARD H. HAUG

November 2015 • Volume 27 • Number 4

ELSEVIER

1600 John F. Kennedy Boulevard • Suite 1800 • Philadelphia, Pennsylvania, 19103-2899

http://www.oralmaxsurgery.theclinics.com

ORAL AND MAXILLOFACIAL SURGERY CLINICS OF NORTH AMERICA Volume 27, Number 4
November 2015 ISSN 1042-3699, ISBN-13: 978-0-323-41346-6

Editor: John Vassallo; j.vassallo@elsevier.com
Developmental Editor: Colleen Viola

Oral and Maxillofacial Surgery Clinics of North America (ISSN 1042-3699) is published quarterly by Elsevier Inc., 360 Park Avenue South, New York, NY 10010-1710. Months of issue are February, May, August, and November. Business and Editorial Offices: 1600 John F. Kennedy Blvd., Suite 1800, Philadelphia, PA 19103-2899. Periodicals postage paid at New York, NY and additional mailing offices. Subscription prices are $385.00 per year for US individuals, $567.00 per year for US institutions, $175.00 per year for US students and residents, $455.00 per year for Canadian individuals, $680.00 per year for Canadian institutions, $520.00 per year for international individuals, $680.00 per year for international institutions and $235.00 per year for Canadian and foreign students/residents. To receive student/resident rate, orders must be accompanied by name or affiliated institution, date of term, and the *signature* of program/residency coordinator on institution letterhead. Orders will be billed at individual rate until proof of status is received. Foreign air speed delivery is included in all *Clinics* subscription prices. All prices are subject to change without notice. **POSTMASTER:** Send address changes to *Oral and Maxillofacial Surgery Clinics of North America,* Elsevier Periodicals **Customer Service, 11830 Westline Industrial Drive, St. Louis, MO 63146. Tel: 1-800-654-2452 (U.S. and Canada); 314-447-8871 (outside U.S. and Canada). Fax: 314-447-8029. E-mail: journals customerservice-usa@elsevier.com (for print support); journalsonlinesupport-usa@elsevier.com (for online support).**

Reprints. For copies of 100 or more, of articles in this publication, please contact the Commercial Reprints Department, Elsevier Inc., 360 Park Avenue South, New York, NY 10010-1710. Tel.: 212-633-3874; Fax: 212-633-3820; Email: reprints@elsevier.com.

Oral and Maxillofacial Surgery Clinics of North America is covered in *MEDLINE/PubMed (Index Medicus)*, *Science Citation Index Expanded (SciSearch®)*, *Journal Citation Reports/Science Edition*, and *Current Contents®/Clinical Medicine*.

Contributors

CONSULTING EDITOR

RICHARD H. HAUG, DDS
Professor and Chief, Oral Maxillofacial Surgery, Carolinas Medical Center, Charlotte, North Carolina

EDITOR

SALVATORE L. RUGGIERO, DMD, MD, FACS
New York Center for Orthognathic and Maxillofacial Surgery, Lake Success; Clinical Professor, Department of Oral and Maxillofacial Surgery, Stony Brook University, Stony Brook; Clinical Professor, Department of Dental Medicine, Hofstra North Shore-LIJ School of Medicine, New Hyde Park, New York

AUTHORS

TARA AGHALOO, DDS, MD, PhD
Professor and Assistant Dean for Clinical Research, Section of Oral and Maxillofacial Surgery, Division of Diagnostic and Surgical Sciences, UCLA School of Dentistry, Los Angeles, California

MATTHEW R. ALLEN, PhD
Associate Professor, Department of Anatomy and Cell Biology, Indiana University School of Medicine, Indianapolis, Indiana

THOMAS B. DODSON, DMD, MPH
Professor and Chair; Associate Dean for Hospital Affairs, Department of Oral and Maxillofacial Surgery, University of Washington School of Dentistry, Seattle, Washington

JOHN E. FANTASIA, DDS
Professor, Division of Oral and Maxillofacial Pathology, Department of Dental Medicine, Hofstra North Shore-LIJ School of Medicine, New Hyde Park, New York

S. FEDELE, DDS, PhD
UCL Eastman Dental Institute, University College London; Biomedical NIHR Research Centre, University College London Hospitals, London, United Kingdom

P.L. FUNG, BDS, MSc, PhD
UCL Eastman Dental Institute, University College London, London, United Kingdom

REGINALD H. GOODDAY, DDS, MSc, FRCD(C), FICD, FACD
Professor, Department of Oral and Maxillofacial Sciences, Faculty of Dentistry, Dalhousie University, Halifax, Nova Scotia, Canada

RENNA HAZBOUN, DMD
Lecturer, Section of Special Patient Care, Division of Advanced Prosthodontics and Section of Restorative Dentistry, Division of Regenerative and Constitutive Sciences, UCLA School of Dentistry, Los Angeles, California

BHOOMI MEHROTRA, MD
Director of Oncology, Department of
Medicine, Cancer Institute at St. Francis
Hospital, The Heart Center, Roslyn,
New York

P. NICOLETTI, MD, PhD
Department of Systems Biology, Irving Cancer
Research Center, Columbia University,
New York, New York

FELICE O'RYAN, DDS
Division Maxillofacial Surgery, Oakland
Medical Center, Kaiser Permanente, Oakland,
California

S. PORTER, MD, PhD, FDS RCS, FDS RCSE
UCL Eastman Dental Institute, University
College London, London, United Kingdom

**SALVATORE L. RUGGIERO, DMD, MD,
FACS**
New York Center for Orthognathic and
Maxillofacial Surgery, Lake Success; Clinical
Professor, Department of Oral and
Maxillofacial Surgery, Stony Brook University,
Stony Brook; Clinical Professor, Department
of Dental Medicine, Hofstra North Shore-LIJ
School of Medicine, New Hyde Park,
New York

Y. SHEN, MD, PhD
Departments of Systems Biology and
Biomedical Informatics, Irving Cancer
Research Center, Columbia University,
New York, New York

SOTIRIOS TETRADIS, DDS, PhD
Professor and Chairman, Section of Oral and
Maxillofacial Radiology, Division of Diagnostic
and Surgical Sciences, UCLA School of
Dentistry; Molecular Biology Institute, UCLA,
Los Angeles, California

GIANINA L. USERA, MD
Endocrinology Fellow, Division of
Endocrinology, Diabetes and Metabolism,
Department of Medicine, Hofstra North
Shore-LIJ School of Medicine, Great Neck,
New York

STUART WEINERMAN, MD
Program Director of Endocrinology Fellowship;
Assistant Professor of Medicine, Division of
Endocrinology, Diabetes and Metabolism,
Department of Medicine, Hofstra North
Shore-LIJ School of Medicine, Great Neck,
New York

WILLIAM BRADFORD WILLIAMS, DMD, MD
Division Maxillofacial Surgery, Oakland
Medical Center, Kaiser Permanente, Oakland,
California

Contents

The relationship between osteonecrosis of the jaw and bisphosphonate therapy was initially established more than 10 years ago. Since that time, our understanding of this disease process has evolved as the direct result of clinical, basic science, and animal research initiatives. Medication-related osteonecrosis of the jaw (MRONJ) is a well-known entity now known to be associated with various antiresorptive therapies and recently with antiangiogenic medications. This article reviews the recently modified diagnostic criteria for MRONJ with a focus on the clinical, histopathologic, and imaging characteristics of this disease process.

Osteonecrosis of the jaw (ONJ) is a multifactorial disease in patients with primary or metastatic bone malignancy or osteoporosis undergoing systemic antiresorptive therapy, where pathophysiology has not yet been fully determined. The staging of ONJ is based on severity of symptoms and extent of clinical and radiographic findings. Treatment strategies range from conservative local wound care to aggressive resective surgery of all necrotic bone. The first ONJ cases were reported in 2003 and 2004, and although significant progress has been made in our understanding of the disease, much more work needs to be done to completely explain its pathophysiology.

In the late 1990s and the early 2000s, bisphosphonates had become the clinical pillar of excellence for treating metabolic bone disease, and thus their connection with osteonecrosis of the jaw (ONJ) caused significant concern. Over the past decade, progress has been made in understanding what is now referred to as medication-related ONJ (MRONJ), because of its connections to agents other than bisphosphonates, although in many respects the progress has been slow. This review highlights the key basic science and translational (animal) studies in the area of MRONJ and suggests areas of focus as the field moves into the next decade.

This article provides the best current frequency estimate of medication-related osteonecrosis of the jaws (MRONJ) and identifies factors associated with the risk of developing osteonecrosis of the jaw (ONJ) among patients exposed to relevant medications (ie, antiresorptive or antiangiogenic agents). MRONJ is a rare but serious complication of cancer treatment or osteoporosis management. This review confirms that antiresorptive medications such as oral or intravenous bisphosphonates and denosumab are the most common risk factors for developing ONJ. The risk of MRONJ is greater in patients with cancer than in those receiving antiresorptive treatments for osteoporosis by a factor of 10.

Medication-related osteonecrosis of the jaw (MRONJ) primarily involves patients receiving intravenous bisphosphonates for treatment of skeletal-related malignancies, oral bisphosphonates, and denosumab. There is no consensus regarding the clinical management of MRONJ. Successful treatment may be that which results in a cure, with complete mucosal coverage and elimination of disease, or that which improves the quality of life without a cure (palliation). Helping patients to understand the chronicity and potential progression of the disease is essential to a satisfactory outcome. This review aims to share our treatment approach to patients with MRONJ. Treatment can be divided into medical and surgical therapies.

For patients at risk of osteonecrosis of the jaw (ONJ), information can be provided by the pharmaceutical manufacturer, pharmacist, prescribing physician, dentist, and oral and maxillofacial surgeon. Prevention strategies to reduce the incidence of osteonecrosis should be applied as soon as it is determined that a patient will be placed on antiresorptive medication. Proper screening involves a comprehensive oral examination with radiographs followed by oral hygiene instruction and necessary dental treatment; surgical techniques and adjunctive therapies that favor optimum healing of bone and soft tissue decrease the risk of ONJ. No dental procedures are absolutely contraindicated.

Osteonecrosis of the jaws (ONJ) is a potentially severe disorder that develops in a subgroup of individuals who have used bisphosphonate (BP) medications. Several clinical risk factors have been associated with the risk of ONJ development, but evidence is limited and in most instances ONJ remains an unpredictable adverse drug reaction. Interindividual genetic variability can contribute to explaining ONJ development in a subset of BP users, and the discovery of relevant associated gene variants could lead to the identification of individuals at higher risk. No genetic variant has been found to be robustly associated with susceptibility to ONJ.

There is an increasing use of established and newer medications that have antiangiogenic properties. Inhibition of angiogenesis likely has either a primary or secondary role in the development of osteonecrosis of the jaw (ONJ). These medications are being used in the treatment of various cancers and in the treatment of several non-oncologic conditions. Antiangiogenic medications, when used in combination with antiresorptive medications such as nitrogen-containing bisphosphonates or denosumab, seem to increase the likelihood of osteonecrosis of the jaw. This review highlights the role of inhibitors of angiogenesis and their role in the development of osteonecrosis of the jaws.

ORAL AND MAXILLOFACIAL SURGERY CLINICS OF NORTH AMERICA

THE CLINICS ARE NOW AVAILABLE ONLINE!
Access your subscription at:
www.theclinics.com

Preface

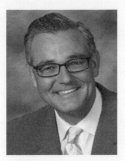

Salvatore L. Ruggiero, DMD, MD, FACS
Editor

Medication-related osteonecrosis of the jaw (MRONJ) that is linked to the treatment of malignant and nonmalignant conditions of the bone continues to receive considerable attention in the scientific and lay community despite the fact that it was initially described over ten years ago. The proven efficacy of antiresorptive agents (bisphosphonates, anti-RANKL antibodies) in the treatment and prevention of skeletally related events will ensure their continued use for the foreseeable future. The more recent reports of jaw necrosis associated with antiangiogenic cancer therapies underscore the complexity of this complication and assure that this entity will remain as one of the more challenging clinical problems for oral and maxillofacial surgeons.

The criteria required to establish the diagnosis of MRONJ as well as the elements of the disease mechanism and the staging system have evolved in order to more accurately reflect the clinical presentation of this disease entity. As the awareness of this complication has grown, so did the realization that more controlled clinical studies and animal research were needed. Research initiatives funded by various government and private institutions provided the necessary support for such studies, and as a result, our knowledge base has certainly increased. In fact, most of the information presented in this issue of *Oral and Maxillofacial Surgery Clinics of North America* stems directly from research endeavors from experts in this field.

In response to our specialty's expanding clinical and research experience in the management of MRONJ, periodic updates are certainly required in order to maintain a proper level of evidenced-based understanding. Jaw necrosis, regardless of the cause, has remained a clinical entity that is typically diagnosed and primarily managed by oral and maxillofacial surgeons, and therefore, it is important for our specialty to remain well informed about all aspects of this disease process, including the drugs responsible for this complication.

The aim of this issue of the *Oral and Maxillofacial Surgery Clinics of North America* is to provide the readership with current information regarding diagnosis, pathophysiology, and strategies for the management and prevention of MRONJ. I am hopeful that this issue will serve as a useful reference for our specialty as the process of evidenced-based learning continues.

Salvatore L. Ruggiero, DMD, MD, FACS
New York Center for Orthognathic and
Maxillofacial Surgery, Lake Success
NY 11042, USA

Department of Oral and Maxillofacial Surgery,
Stony Brook University, Stony Brook
NY 11794, USA

Department of Dental Medicine, Hofstra North
Shore-LIJ School of Medicine, New Hyde Park
NY 11040, USA

E-mail address:
sruggie@optonline.net

Oral Maxillofacial Surg Clin N Am 27 (2015) ix
http://dx.doi.org/10.1016/j.coms.2015.08.005
1042-3699/15/$ – see front matter © 2015 Published by Elsevier Inc.

Diagnosis and Staging of Medication-Related Osteonecrosis of the Jaw

Salvatore L. Ruggiero, DMD, MD[a,b,*]

KEYWORDS

- Osteonecrosis • Medication-related osteonecrosis of the jaw • Jaw necrosis
- Antiresorptive therapy • Antiangiogenic therapy

KEY POINTS

- The association of antiangiogenic therapy with osteonecrosis of the jaw has prompted a change in nomenclature to medication-related osteonecrosis of the jaw (MRONJ).
- The diagnostic criteria for MRONJ has expanded to include fistulas that can be probed to bone.
- The imaging characteristics of MRONJ are helpful in defining the extent of the process but are not diagnostic.
- Obtaining a complete patient history and clinical examination remains the most effective mode of establishing a diagnosis of MRONJ.
- Proper staging of MRONJ is essential for directing stage-specific treatment guidelines.

INTRODUCTION

Medication-related osteonecrosis of the jaw (MRONJ) is now a well-known complication associated with antiresorptive and antiangiogenic therapies that is affecting a growing number of patients. In response to our specialty's expanding clinical experience in the management of MRONJ, updated treatment guidelines were required in 2009 and most recently in 2014. MRONJ patients often present with challenging clinical problems requiring varying degrees of intervention and oral and maxillofacial surgical care. Stage-specific treatment protocols have been created, and recently modified, to guide oral surgeons and other health care professionals in selecting the appropriate operative or nonoperative treatment strategy. Establishing the correct diagnosis and properly stratifying these patients is crucial in providing necessary care in a timely fashion. Moreover, this approach will permit us to guide our medical and dental colleagues, who will often modify the patient management plan if a diagnosis of MRONJ is suspected.

The aim of this article is to review the recently modified diagnostic criteria for MRONJ with a focus on the clinical, histopathologic, and imaging characteristics of this disease process. Elements of the staging criteria are also examined along with the rationale for the various changes that been implemented since the original American Association of Oral and Maxillofacial Surgeons (AAOMS) position paper in 2007.

NOMENCLATURE AND DIAGNOSTIC CRITERIA

Standardization of diagnostic criteria and nomenclature for this clinical entity is important to

---

Disclosure: Consultant for Amgen Inc.

[a] Department of Oral and Maxillofacial Surgery, School of Dental Medicine, SUNY, Stony Brook, NY 11794-8705, USA; [b] Hofstra North Shore - LIJ School of Medicine, Division of Oral and Maxillofacial Surgery, 270-05 76th Ave, New Hyde park, New York, NY 11040, USA
* Corresponding author. New York Center for Orthognathic and Maxillofacial Surgery, 2001 Marcus Avenue, Suite N10, Lake Success, NY 11042.
E-mail address: drruggiero@nycoms.com

Oral Maxillofacial Surg Clin N Am 27 (2015) 479–487
http://dx.doi.org/10.1016/j.coms.2015.06.008

facilitate future clinical and epidemiologic research. In addition, a uniform definition for osteonecrosis of the jaw (ONJ) will serve to distinguish this new clinical entity from other delayed intraoral healing conditions. Since it was first described, various organizations have proposed clinical definitions for ONJ, all of which are analogous to each other; and this has resulted in some degree of confusion. This condition is known in the literature by several acronyms, including BRONJ (bisphosphonate-related osteonecrosis of the jaw), BRON (bisphosphonate-related osteonecrosis), BON (bisphosphonate osteonecrosis), BAONJ (bisphosphonate-associated osteonecrosis of the jaw), and simply ONJ. The emergence of jaw necrosis in bisphosphonate-naïve patients receiving monoclonal therapy with RANKL inhibitors[1-4] prompted the American Dental Association to introduce the more generic term ARONJ (antiresorptive-associated osteonecrosis of the jaw).[5] MRONJ (medication-related osteonecrosis of the jaw) is the most recent nomenclature change that was proposed in the current AAOMS position paper.[6] This modification, though broad in its scope, was considered necessary to address the growing number of osteonecrosis cases affecting jaws that were associated with antiangiogenic therapies.

Despite the variations in nomenclature, the clinical finding of exposed, necrotic bone remains the consistent hallmark of the diagnosis; therefore, a physical examination is the most effective method of establishing the diagnosis of jaw necrosis.

The AAOMS established a working definition for MRONJ since it was first defined in 2006. The recent position paper contained 2 modifications to the definition. More specifically, antiangiogenic agents were added to the list of medications, and "bone that can be probed" was considered equivalent to exposed bone. These changes were implemented so that MRONJ could be more accurately distinguished from other delayed healing conditions and address evolving clinical observations and concerns about underreporting of disease. A diagnosis of MRONJ should be considered if a patient presents with all of the following criteria:

1. Current or previous treatment with antiresorptive and/or antiangiogenic agents
2. Exposed bone or bone that can be probed through an intraoral or extraoral fistula(e) in the maxillofacial region that has persisted for more than 8 weeks
3. No history of radiation therapy to the jaws or obvious metastatic disease to the jaws

The differential diagnosis of MRONJ should exclude other common clinical conditions such as alveolar osteitis, sinusitis, gingivitis/periodontitis, periapical disorder, and temporomandibular joint disorders. In those rare situations where exposed bone is present in patients exposed to bisphosphonates and radiation therapy to the jaw, osteoradionecrosis should be strongly considered. Although bone inflammation and infection is typically present in patients with advanced MRONJ, this is typically a secondary event. The exposed bone and surrounding soft tissue become secondarily infected, presenting a clinical scenario similar to that of osteomyelitis. However, the histologic analysis of these bone specimens rarely demonstrates the criteria required to establish a diagnosis of acute or chronic osteomyelitis. Analyses of the physical properties of the resected necrotic bone have also failed to demonstrate any unique features that would serve as a reliable biomarker for this disease process.[7,8] A heightened level of awareness for MRONJ should exist among patients with cancer receiving antiresorptive or antiangiogenic medication, as these patients are significantly more likely than those with osteoporosis to develop this complication.[6,9]

CLINICAL PRESENTATION

The patient's history and clinical examination continues to be the most sensitive diagnostic tools for this condition. Obtaining an accurate exposure history to the various antiresorptive and antiangiogenic medications is a critical first step in assessing for MRONJ. Cancer and non-cancer patients will often present with complicated antiresorptive medication schedules as their physicians attempt to modulate therapy according to disease activity and risk. Patients are often unaware of the specific type of medications they are receiving, especially patients with cancer who are typically receiving multiple chemotherapy medications.[10] For the clinician evaluating these patients, it is important to obtain an accurate assessment of the continuous total drug-exposure history because often there will be a hiatus in therapy (intentional or because of noncompliance) that will affect the probability of establishing a diagnosis of MRONJ. Reviewing the medication history with the treating oncologist or endocrinologist is often required to obtain the necessary information.

Regions of exposed and necrotic bone may remain asymptomatic for weeks, months, or even years. These lesions are most frequently symptomatic when surrounding tissues become inflamed or there is clinical evidence of exposed bone. Signs and symptoms that may occur before the development of clinically detectable osteonecrosis include pain, tooth mobility, mucosal swelling, erythema, and ulceration. These symptoms may occur spontaneously or, more commonly, at the site of prior dentoalveolar surgery, which continues to be a major risk factor for this process. Recent controlled studies have reported a 16- to 33-fold increased risk of MRONJ associated with extractions in patients with cancer receiving antiresorptive therapy.[11–13] However, it has also been reported in patients with no history of trauma or in edentulous regions of the jaw. Intraoral and extraoral fistulae may develop when necrotic jawbone becomes secondarily infected. Some patients may also present with complaints of altered sensation in the affected area as the neurovascular bundle becomes compressed from the inflamed surrounding bone. Chronic maxillary sinusitis secondary to osteonecrosis with or without an oral-antral fistula can be the presenting symptom in patients with maxillary bone involvement that extends to the sinus floor (**Fig. 1**).

Recent controlled studies have supported prior case series, which reported that MRONJ lesions are found more commonly in the mandible than the maxilla. In a study by Saad and colleagues,[12] 73% of cancer patients with bone metastases presented with mandibular MRONJ while 22% had maxillary involvement. Lesions are also more prevalent in areas with thin mucosa overlying bone prominences such as tori, exostoses, and the myelohyoid ridge.[14,15] These observations are supported by other studies that report an increased incidence of MRONJ in patients with cancer who are denture wearers.[13,16]

The size of the affected area can be variable, and range from a nonhealing extraction site to exposure and necrosis of large sections of jawbone. The area of exposed bone is typically surrounded by inflamed erythematous soft tissue. Purulent discharge at the site of exposed bone will be present when these sites become secondarily infected. Microbial cultures from areas of exposed bone will usually demonstrate a polymicrobial infection populated with normal oral microbes. Culture data have not consistently identified specific pathogens related to this disease process. Therefore, a diagnosis of microbial infection requires confirmation with microbial cultures, and should not be made solely on histologic identification of bacterial debris. The development of biofilms adherent to the surface of exposed necrotic bone involves complex multiorganism colonies that have been well described and may account for the poor response to systemic antimicrobial therapy in certain patients.[17–20] In cases where there is extensive soft-tissue involvement, however, microbial culture data may define comorbid oral infections that may facilitate the selection of an appropriate antibiotic regimen.

IMAGING

The radiographic features of MRONJ remain relatively nonspecific. In fact, plain film radiography does not typically demonstrate any abnormality in the early stages of the disease because of the limited degree of decalcification that is present, and therefore are poor screening tools for this entity. However, findings on plain film imaging such as localized or diffuse osteosclerosis or a thickening of the lamina dura may be predictors for future sites of exposed, necrotic bone. Little or no ossification at a previous extraction site may also represent an early radiographic sign (**Fig. 2**). The findings on computed tomography (CT) are also nonspecific, but this modality is significantly more sensitive to changes in bone mineralization, and therefore is more likely to demonstrate areas of focal sclerosis, thickened lamina dura, early sequestrum formation, and the presence of reactive periosteal bone (**Fig. 3**).[21]

CT images have also proved to be more accurate in delineating the extent of disease, which is

Fig. 1. Coronal cone-beam scan in a patient with stage 3 MRONJ. There is partial opacification of the right maxillary sinus, with sequestration of the maxillary alveolar bone extending to the sinus floor (*arrow*).

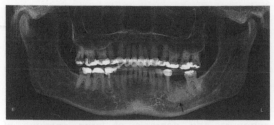

Fig. 2. Panoramic radiograph demonstrating a focal osteosclerosis, delayed healing at extraction site, and poor ossification (*arrow*) in a patient with multiple myeloma and 3-year history of intravenous zoledronate therapy. The tooth had been extracted 3 years before this radiograph was taken.

helpful for surgical treatment planning.[22,23] It is the observation of this author that cases of MRONJ associated with antiangiogenic therapy may differ from other cases in that the basilar bone seems to be more frequently affected (**Fig. 4**). Technetium-99m bone scanning is a highly sensitive imaging modality for the identification of inflammation, which is commonly present in patients with established MRONJ. The utility of bone scintigraphy in patients at risk of MRONJ has received growing attention following reports of increased tracer

uptake in regions of the jaws that subsequently developed necrosis.[24,25] Although nuclear imaging has limited value in patients with existing disease because of its poor specificity, its usefulness as a predictive tool in patients with preclinical disease (stage 0) seems to have some level of theoretic benefit and therefore requires continued evaluation. MRI is also a highly sensitive imaging modality for the presence of osseous edema and inflammation, and is often used to identify the early acute phase of osteomyelitis. The imaging characteristics of MRI in patients with MRONJ have been described.[26,27] However, owing to its low level of specificity it has limited predictive value for detecting early disease. A recent retrospective study analyzed the utility of PET in MRONJ patients with established disease and reported a low level of sensitivity, specificity, and accuracy, implying limited diagnostic value for this imaging modality.[28]

HISTOPATHOLOGY

The histologic presentation of MRONJ specimens has been well described by Fantasia.[29] In gross terms, MRONJ specimens are composed of gray-tan hard tissue with or without fragmented

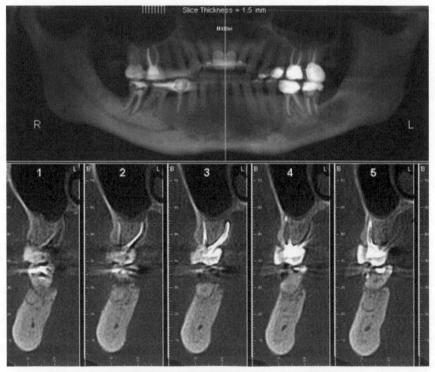

Fig. 3. Diffuse osteosclerosis and widening of the periodontal ligament space of the mandibular body in a patient with multiple myeloma and a history of intravenous zoledronate therapy.

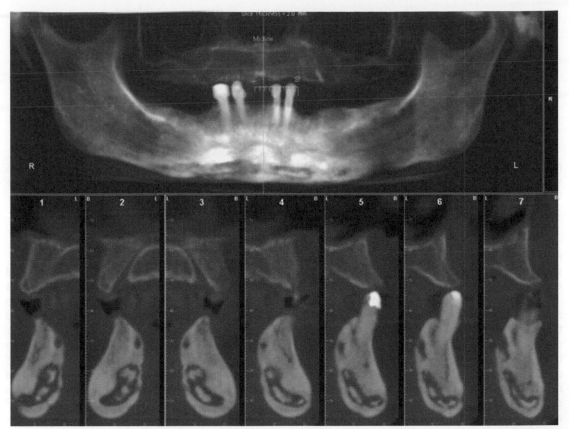

Fig. 4. Cone-beam scan of a 53-year-old patient who was receiving antiangiogenic therapy for the treatment of a malignant gastrointestinal stromal tumor. Sequestration of the intramedullary basilar bone is noted in the anterior mandible along with osteosclerosis and extraoral fistula formation. This patient had no history of local trauma or dentoalveolar surgery.

friable soft tissue. Large specimens can require significant decalcification times in acidic solutions, a testament to the sclerotic nature of the involved bone. In a study by Allen and colleagues,[8] necrotic bone samples from patients with established MRONJ were analyzed with high-resolution micro-CT and compared with cadaver controls. The density values for MRONJ samples demonstrated a high degree of heterogeneity, suggesting that density measurements may have limitations as a biomarker for early detection of this condition. Some smaller bone specimens may have a soft consistency, possibly the result of bacterial acids resulting in demineralization in vivo. Debridement specimens, sequestra, and resection specimens of MRONJ are all similar histologically (**Fig. 5**). Necrotic bone characterized by absence of osteocytes is the hallmark of this entity. The bone is invariably sclerotic and, if exposed to the oral cavity, will have bacterial debris adherent to the necrotic bone surface. Osteoclasts are typically

absent, a finding that may be reflective of osteoclast apoptosis caused by the antiresorptive agent. Adjacent soft tissues typically consist of granulation tissue with or without abscess formation. Although the histologic characteristics of MRONJ specimens may not be pathognomonic for this disease process, the importance of a histologic analysis is underscored by a recent study reporting cancer in these bone specimens.[30] In this retrospective cohort multicenter study, the histologic analysis of 357 sites of suspected MRONJ revealed metastatic cancer or multiple myeloma in 5% of the specimens.

CLINICAL STAGING

A clinical staging system developed by Ruggiero and colleagues,[15] and adopted by the AAOMS in 2006[31] and updated in 2009[32] and 2014,[6] has served to categorize patients with MRONJ, direct rational treatment guidelines, and collect data to

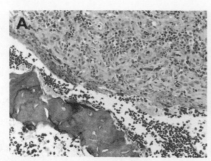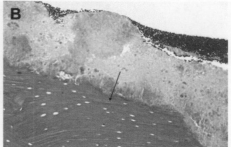

Fig. 5. (*A*) Necrotic bone (*arrow*) characterized by lacunae devoid of osteocytes. Microorganisms are noted on the surface of the necrotic bone (hematoxylin-eosin, original magnification ×200). (*B*) Sequestrum of necrotic bone (*arrow*) and adjacent granulation tissue (hematoxylin-eosin, original magnification ×400).

assess the prognosis and treatment outcomes in patients who have used either antiresorptive or antiangiogenic medications (**Table 1**).

Patients with no evidence of exposed or necrotic bone are considered to be "at risk" if they have been exposed to either antiresorptive or antiangiogenic medications. The potency of the antiresorptive used, the duration of exposure, and recent dentoalveolar surgery seem to be the main determinants in assessing the risk of developing ONJ. The risk associated with targeted antiangiogenic cancer therapies (vascular endothelial growth factor and tyrosine kinase inhibitors) are also associated with jaw necrosis, but further studies of these medications are warranted to assess risk stratification.

In the 2009 AAOMS guidelines, a stage 0 category was created to segregate "at risk" patients with nonspecific signs and symptoms such as

pain, abscess formation, altered sensory function, or osteosclerosis, but with no clinical evidence of necrosis or exposed bone (see **Fig. 2**). Since then, several cases studies have reported that up to 50% of patients with stage 0 have progressed to stages 1, 2, or 3.[25,33]

The 2014 AAOMS guidelines redefined this category as "stage 0 (nonexposed bone variant)" to accommodate additional radiographic signs and address growing concerns that this stage is a real precursor for clinical disease (**Box 1**).[32] The degree to which patients with stage 0 (nonexposed bone variant) disease progress to overt ONJ remains to be furthered clarified, and therefore represents an important area for future investigation.

Patients with stage 1 disease have exposed and necrotic bone or fistula that probes to bone, but are asymptomatic and have no evidence of

Table 1 MRONJ staging	
At risk category	No apparent exposed/necrotic bone in patients who have been treated with either antiresorptive or antiangiogenic agents
Stage 0	Nonspecific clinical findings and symptoms such as jaw pain or osteosclerosis but no clinical evidence of exposed bone (see **Box 1**)
Stage 1	Exposed, necrotic bone or fistula that probes to bone No symptoms or evidence of infection
Stage 2	Exposed, necrotic bone or fistula that probes to bone, associated with infection, pain, and erythema in the regions of the exposed bone Purulent drainage may also be present
Stage 3	Exposed, necrotic bone or fistula that probes to bone in patients with pain, infection, and 1 or more of the following: pathologic fracture, extraoral fistula, oral antral/oral nasal communication or osteolysis extending to the inferior border or sinus floor

From Ruggiero S, Fantasia J, Carlson E. Bisphosphonate-related osteonecrosis of the jaw: background and guidelines for diagnosis, staging and management. Oral Surg Oral Med Oral Pathol Oral Radiol Endod 2006;102:436; with permission.

Box 1
Stage 0 (nonexposed bone variant)

Definition

- Patients with no clinical evidence of necrotic bone, but who present with nonspecific symptoms or clinical and radiographic findings, such as:

Symptoms

- Odontalgia not explained by an odontogenic cause
- Dull, aching bone pain in the jaw, which may radiate to the temporomandibular joint region
- Sinus pain, which may be associated with inflammation and thickening of the maxillary sinus wall
- Altered neurosensory function

Clinical Findings

- Loosening of teeth not explained by chronic periodontal disease
- Periapical/periodontal fistula that is not associated with pulpal necrosis attributed to caries, trauma, or restorations

Radiographic Findings

- Alveolar bone loss or resorption not attributable to chronic periodontal disease
- Changes to trabecular pattern: dense bone and no new bone in extraction sockets
- Regions of osteosclerosis involving the alveolar bone and/or the surrounding basilar bone
- Thickening/obscuring of periodontal ligament (thickening of the lamina dura, sclerosis, and decreased size of the periodontal ligament space)

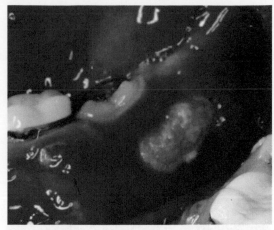

Fig. 7. Stage 2 MRONJ. Clinical photo of exposed bone along the lingual plate region that is associated with surrounding soft-tissue infection and fistula formation (*arrow*). Arrow is present and depicts the fistula.

infection (**Fig. 6**). In addition to exposed bone, these patients may also present with radiographic findings mentioned for stage 0 (nonexposed bone variant), which are localized to the alveolar bone region.

There is no evidence of significant adjacent or regional soft-tissue inflammatory swelling or infection. It is possible that patients may have symptoms of pain before the development of radiographic changes that are suspicious for osteonecrosis or exposed bone.

Stage 2 disease is characterized by exposed and necrotic bone, or fistula that probes to bone, with evidence of infection (**Fig. 7**). Patients with stage 2 disease are typically symptomatic and present with pain, adjacent or regional soft-tissue inflammatory swelling, or secondary infection. These patients may also present with radiographic findings mentioned for stage 0 (nonexposed bone variant) within the alveolar bone region.

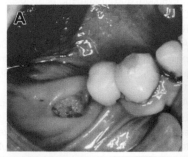
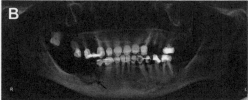

Fig. 6. (*A*) Stage 1 MRONJ. Clinical photo of exposed bone at the right posterior mandible in a 63-year-old man with a history of metastatic prostate cancer and denosumab therapy. (*B*) Stage 1 MRONJ. Panoramic radiograph demonstrating a well-delineated sequestrum (*arrow*) localized to the alveolar bone.

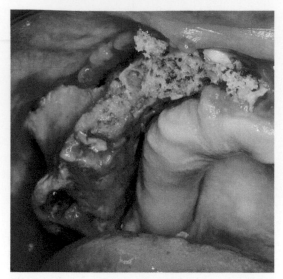

Fig. 8. Stage 3 MRONJ. Clinical photo of exposed and necrotic right maxillary bone. The area of necrosis extends to the midportion of the posterior maxillary buttress (see the corresponding radiograph in **Fig. 1**).

Patients with stage 3 disease (**Figs. 8** and **9**) have exposed and necrotic bone, or fistulae that probe to bone, with evidence of infection associated with pain, adjacent or regional soft-tissue inflammatory swelling, or secondary infection, in addition to 1 or more of the following:

- Exposed necrotic bone extending beyond the region of alveolar bone, that is, inferior border and ramus in the mandible, maxillary sinus, and zygoma in the maxilla
- Pathologic fracture
- Extraoral fistula
- Oral-antral/oral nasal communication
- Osteolysis extending to the inferior border of the mandible or sinus floor

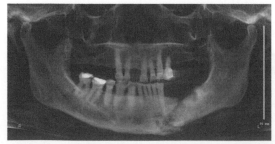

Fig. 9. Stage 3 MRONJ. Pathologic fracture of the left mandible in a 68-year-old man who was receiving intravenous antiresorptive therapy for multiple myeloma.

SUMMARY

Our understanding of the pathogenesis of MRONJ and how it influences the clinical presentation continues to evolve. The numerous imaging modalities that have been used to evaluate MRONJ have served as useful adjunctive tools in assessing the extent of disease or planning operative treatment. However, they have not provided the degree of specificity to be considered a valid diagnostic tool. The histologic features of MRONJ samples are often supportive of the diagnosis, but are rarely pathognomonic and are often difficult to differentiate from other inflammatory bone conditions. Obtaining a complete patient history and clinical examination remains the most effective mode of establishing a timely diagnosis of MRONJ in most patients. The patient history, imaging data, and histopathology provide the supportive elements to establish the diagnosis of MRONJ when a patient presents with exposed and necrotic jawbone. This approach will facilitate proper disease stratification and implementation of stage-specific treatment strategies.

REFERENCES

1. Lipton A, Fizazi K, Stopeck AT, et al. Superiority of denosumab to zoledronic acid for prevention of skeletal-related events: a combined analysis of 3 pivotal, randomised, phase 3 trials. Eur J Cancer 2012; 48(16):3082–92.
2. Aghaloo T, Felsenfeld A, Tetradis S. Osteonecrosis of the jaw in a patient on denosumab. J Oral Maxillofac Surg 2010;68:959–63.
3. Taylor K, Middlefell L, Mizen K. Osteonecrosis of the jaws induced by anti-RANK ligand therapy. Br J Oral Maxillofac Surg 2010;48:221–3.
4. Diz P, Lopez-Cedrun J, Arenaz J, et al. Denasumab-related osteonecrosis of the jaw. J Am Dent Assoc 2012;143(9):981–4.
5. Hellstein J, Adler R, Edwards B, et al. Managing the care of patients receiving antiresorptive therapy for prevention and treatment of osteoporosis. J Am Dent Assoc 2011;142(11):1243–51.
6. Ruggiero S, Dodson T, Fantasia J, et al. American Association of Oral and Maxillofacial Surgeons paper on medication-related osteonecrosis of the jaw—2014 update. J Oral Maxillofac Surg 2014;72: 1938–56.
7. Allen M, Pandya B, Ruggiero S. Lack of correlation between duration of osteonecrosis of the jaw and sequestra tissue morphology: what it tells us about the condition and what it means for future studies. J Oral Maxillofac Surg 2010;68:2730–4.
8. Allen M, Ruggiero S. Higher bone matrix density exists in only a subset of patients with

bisphosphonate-related osteonecrosis of the jaw. J Oral Maxillofac Surg 2009;67:1373–7.

9. Henry D, Costa L, Goldwasser F, et al. A double-blind, randomized study of denosumab versus zolendronic acid for the treatment of bone metastases in patients with advanced cancer (excluding breast and prostate) or multiple myeloma. J Clin Oncol 2011;29:1125.

10. Migliorati C, Mattos K, Palazzolo M. How patients' lack of knowledge about oral bisphosphonates can interfere with medical and dental care. J Am Dent Assoc 2010;141:562–6.

11. Fehm T, Beck V, Banys M, et al. Bisphosphonate-related osteonecrosis of the jaws: incidence and risk factors in patients with breast cancer and gynecological malignancies. Gynecol Oncol 2009;112(3): 605–9.

12. Saad F, Brown JE, Van Poznak C, et al. Incidence, risk factors, and outcomes of osteonecrosis of the jaw: integrated analysis from three blinded active-controlled phase III trials in cancer patients with bone metastases. Ann Oncol 2012;23(5):1341–7.

13. Vahtsevanos K, Kyrgidis A, Verrou E. Longitudinal cohort study of risk factors in cancer patients with bisphosphonate-related osteonecrosis of the jaw. J Clin Oncol 2009;27(32):5356–62.

14. Marx R, Sawatari Y, Fortin M. Bisphosphonate-induced exposed bone (osteonecrosis/osteopetrosis) of the jaws: risk factors, recognition, prevention and treatment. J Oral Maxillofac Surg 2005;63: 1567–75.

15. Ruggiero S, Fantasia J, Carlson E. Bisphosphonate-related osteonecrosis of the jaw: background and guidelines for diagnosis, staging and management. Oral Surg Oral Med Oral Pathol Oral Radiol Endod 2006;102:433–41.

16. Kyrgidis A, Vahtsevanos K, Koloutsos G. Bisphosphonate-related osteonecrosis of the jaws: a case controlled study of risk factors in breast cancer patients. J Clin Oncol 2008;26(28):4634–8.

17. Kumar S, Gorur A, Schaudinn C, et al. The role of microbial biofilms in osteonecrosis of the jaw associated with bisphosphonate therapy. Curr Osteoporos Rep 2010;8(1):40–8 (1544-2241 (Electronic)).

18. Sedghizadeh P, Kumar S, Gorur A, et al. Identification of microbial biofilms in osteonecrosis of the jaws secondary to bisphosphonate therapy. J Oral Maxillofac Surg 2008;66:767–75.

19. Sedghizadeh PP, Stanley K, Caligiuri M, et al. Oral bisphosphonate use and the prevalence of osteonecrosis of the jaw: an institutional inquiry. J Am Dent Assoc 2009;140(1):61–6.

20. Wanger G, Gorby Y, El-Naggar M, et al. Electrically conductive bacterial nanowires in bisphosphonate-related osteonecrosis of the jaw biofilms. Oral Surg Oral Med Oral Pathol Oral Radiol Endod 2013;115: 71–8.

21. Bianchi S, Scoletta M, Cassione F, et al. Computerized tomographic findings in bisphosphonate-associated osteonecrosis of the jaw in patients with cancer. Oral Surg Oral Med Oral Pathol Oral Radiol Endod 2007;104:249–58.

22. Treister N, Friedland B, Woo S. Use of cone-beam computerized tomography for evaluation of bisphosphonate-associated osteonecrosis of the jaws. Oral Surg Oral Med Oral Pathol Oral Radiol Endod 2010;109:753–64.

23. Arce K, Assael L, Weissman J, et al. Image findings in bisphosphonate-related osteonecrosis of the jaws. J Oral Maxillofac Surg 2009;67(Suppl 1):75–84.

24. Chiandussi S, Biasotto M, Cavalli F, et al. Clinical and diagnostic imaging of bisphosphonate-associated osteonecrosis of the jaws. Dentomaxillofac Radiol 2006;35:236–43.

25. O'Ryan F, Khoury S, Liao W, et al. Intravenous bisphosphonate-related osteonecrosis of the jaw: bone scintigraphy as an early indicator. J Oral Maxillofac Surg 2009;67:1363–72.

26. Bedogni A, Blandamura S, Lokmic Z, et al. Bisphosphonate-associated jawbone osteonecrosis: a correlation between imaging techniques and histopathology. Oral Surg Oral Med Oral Pathol Oral Radiol Endod 2008;105(3):358–64.

27. Garcia-Ferrer L, Bagan JV, Martinez-Sanjuan V, et al. MRI of mandibular osteonecrosis secondary to bisphosphonates. Am J Roentgenol 2008;190(4): 949–55.

28. Belcher R, Boyette J, Pierson T, et al. What is the role of positron emission tomography in osteonecrosis of the jaws? J Oral Maxillofac Surg 2014;72(2):306–10.

29. Fantasia JE. Bisphosphonates—what the dentist needs to know: practical considerations. J Oral Maxillofac Surg 2009;67(5):53–60.

30. Carlson ER, Fleisher KE, Ruggiero SL. Metastatic cancer identified in osteonecrosis specimens of the jaws in patients receiving intravenous bisphosphonate medications. J Oral Maxillofac Surg 2013;71(12):2077–86.

31. Advisory Task Force on Bisphosphonate-Related Osteonecrosis of the Jaws, American Association of Oral and Maxillofacial Surgeons. American Association of Oral and Maxillofacial Surgeons position paper on bisphosphonate-related osteonecrosis of the jaw. J Oral Maxillofac Surg 2007;3:369–76.

32. Ruggiero S, Dodson T, Assael L, et al. American Association of Oral and Maxillofacial Surgeons position paper on bisphosphonate-related osteonecrosis of the jaws: 2009 update. J Oral Maxillofac Surg 2009;67:2–12.

33. Fedele S, Porter S, D'Aiuto F, et al. Nonexposed variant of bisphosphonate-associated osteonecrosis of the jaw: a case series. Am J Med 2010; 123:1060–4.

Pathophysiology of Osteonecrosis of the Jaws

Tara Aghaloo, DDS, MD, PhD[a],*, Renna Hazboun, DMD[b], Sotirios Tetradis, DDS, PhD[c,d]

KEYWORDS

- Osteonecrosis of the jaws (ONJ) • Bisphosphonates • MRONJ • Antiresorptive • Pathophysiology

KEY POINTS

- Osteonecrosis of the jaw (ONJ) is a multifactorial disease in patients with primary or metastatic bone malignancy or osteoporosis undergoing systemic antiresorptive therapy, where the pathophysiology has not yet been fully determined.
- The staging of ONJ is based on severity of symptoms and extent of clinical and radiographic findings.
- Treatment strategies range from conservative local wound care to aggressive resective surgery of all necrotic bone.
- The first ONJ cases were reported in 2003 and 2004, and although significant progress has been made in our understanding of the disease, much more work needs to be done to completely explain its pathophysiology.

INTRODUCTION

Osteonecrosis of the jaw (ONJ) was defined as exposed, necrotic bone in the maxillofacial region for at least 8 weeks in patients receiving an antiresorptive medication for primary or metastatic bone cancer, osteoporosis, or Paget disease, without history of radiation therapy to the jaws.[1,2] Recently, the American Association of Oral and Maxillofacial Surgeons (AAOMS) revised the definition to include exposed bone, or bone that can be probed through an intraoral or extraoral fistula in patients on antiresorptive or antiangiogenic medications.[3] The addition of "probed bone" to the case definition is of clinical significance because frank exposed bone is not always seen, even though it is notably necrotic and radiographically similar.

The staging of the disease is based on severity of symptoms and extent of clinical and radiographic findings.[3] The 2009 and 2014 AAOMS position papers outline the disease stages including stage 0, where there is no frank bone exposure.[2,3] Chronic exposed, necrotic bone, inflammation, swelling, pain, and radiographic changes are some of the more common clinical findings. ONJ can present as subtle, commonly overlooked stage 0; as exposed bone without any pain or signs of infection (stage 1); as exposed bone with associated infection, pain, or swelling (stage 2); or as extensive disease that forms in large segments of the maxilla or mandible with extraoral fistulae, involvement of vital structures, or pathologic fracture (stage 3).

Treatment strategies range from conservative local wound care to aggressive resective surgery

a Section of Oral and Maxillofacial Surgery, Division of Diagnostic and Surgical Sciences, UCLA School of Dentistry, 10833 Le Conte Ave., Los Angeles, CA 90095-1668, USA; b Section of Special Patient Care, Division of Advanced Prosthodontics and Section of Restorative Dentistry, Division of Regenerative and Constitutive Sciences, UCLA School of Dentistry, 10833 Le Conte Ave., Los Angeles, CA 90095-1668, USA; c Section of Oral and Maxillofacial Radiology, Division of Diagnostic and Surgical Sciences, UCLA School of Dentistry, 10833 Le Conte Ave., Los Angeles, CA 90095-1668, USA; d Molecular Biology Institute, UCLA, Los Angeles, CA 90095, USA
* Corresponding author.
E-mail address: taghaloo@dentistry.ucla.edu

Oral Maxillofacial Surg Clin N Am 27 (2015) 489–496
http://dx.doi.org/10.1016/j.coms.2015.06.001
1042-3699/15/$ – see front matter © 2015 Elsevier Inc. All rights reserved.

of all necrotic bone. Conservative strategies include systemic antibiotics, oral antibacterial rinse, and debridement of loose necrotic bone that no longer has soft tissue coverage. Recent literature demonstrates that disease prevention with dental examinations and treatment before initiating antiresorptive therapy is the most effective method to decrease ONJ incidence.[4] In the conservative management of patients with active ONJ, the treatment goal is focused on preventing disease progression rather than reversal of the process.[4–7] Any procedures that remove soft tissue and/or expose bone, including extractions, are generally avoided when a conservative treatment plan is followed. More invasive treatment strategies may include local curettage and debridement, en bloc resection, flap advancement, and resective surgery.[8–10]

PROPOSED HYPOTHESES OF MEDICATION-RELATED OSTEONECROSIS OF THE JAW PATHOPHYSIOLOGY

The first ONJ cases were reported in 2003 and 2004, and although significant progress has been made in our understanding of the disease, much more work needs to be done to completely explain its pathophysiology.[11,12] Many hypotheses have been proposed, which have sparked empirically based treatment modalities. Because it is unlikely that one single hypothesis can explain the pathophysiology of ONJ, as it is indeed multifactorial, it is also unlikely that one treatment modality will be successful in all patients. Moreover, because ONJ is a relatively newly described disease entity, as more clinical and preclinical evidence becomes available, it is apparent that our hypotheses and treatment approaches will need to be continuously modified.

Hypothesis 1: Bone-Remodeling Inhibition

Osteoclast activity is tightly regulated by receptor activator of nuclear factor kappa B (RANK)/RANK ligand (RANKL)/osteoprotegerin (OPG) signaling, where an increase in RANKL or decrease in OPG lead to increased bone resorption. In cancer states, tumor cells release growth factors or cytokines, which in turn stimulate osteoblast RANKL release, causing increased bone resorption, and subsequently increased tumor cell presence and growth.[13] Because of their direct effects on osteoclasts, antiresorptives significantly decrease skeletal-related complications, relieve severe bone pain, and correct hypercalcemia in patients with malignant diseases.[14–18]

Bisphosphonates (BPs) have direct effects on osteoclasts to significantly attenuate bone remodeling[19,20] and decrease skeletal-related complications in patients with malignant diseases or osteoporosis.[14,15,20] Osteoclast differentiation and function play vital roles in bone healing and remodeling at all skeletal sites, but ONJ occurs only in alveolar bone of the maxilla and mandible.[21] Alveolar bone may demonstrate an increased remodeling rate as compared with other bones in the axial or appendicular skeleton, which may explain the ONJ predilection in the jaws.[22,23] However, other studies have failed to confirm differences in bone turnover between the mandible and femur by bone scintigraphy; although the maxilla did show increased bone turnover, administration of BP or denosumab did not change the turnover rate of any bones.[24] Interestingly in mice, fluorescent-labeled BPs demonstrate preferential accumulation in sites of tooth extraction or dental disease, where bone turnover is increased. This is why increased uptake may predispose such sites to higher BP doses and increase susceptibility to BP effects. Although this may not demonstrate a general increase in bone turnover in the jaws, it does show a localized increase in potentially future ONJ sites.[25] The increased bone resorption in the setting of dental disease, coupled with the thin overlying mucosa and a direct pathway through the periodontal ligament with the external environment, make the jaws a suitable breeding ground for ONJ to develop.

Because the primary mechanism of BPs and denosumab is to inhibit osteoclast function by different mechanisms, it is not surprising that altered bone remodeling is the leading hypothesis for ONJ development.[26–29] Importantly, the prevalence of ONJ in patients receiving denosumab and BPs is not significantly different.[30–32] Moreover, animal studies demonstrate a similar rate of periosteal bone deposition, histologic necrosis, and bone exposure when rodents with periodontal or periapical disease or tooth extractions are treated with zoledronate as compared with RANKL inhibitors.[21,33–35] These human and animal studies highlight the central role of bone remodeling suppression. To combat the effects of bone turnover suppression, withdrawing antiresorptive medications before tooth extraction of surgical procedures is often advocated to potentially reduce the risk of ONJ[3,36–38]; however, no controlled studies confirm the reduction or reversal of ONJ after a "drug holiday." Only one clinical report demonstrates a 40% resolution after discontinuing denosumab and 30% after discontinuing zoledronic acid (ZA).[31]

ONJ prevalence in patients treated with BP or denosumab appears similar.[39,40] BPs bind to exposed hydroxyapatite and incorporate into the bone matrix, where they are retained with a half-life of many years.[41-43] With the advent of denosumab, which does not incorporate into the bone matrix, the half-life is significantly shorter at 32 days maximum[44,45] and rapid reversibility of its antiresorptive effects.[46] Interestingly, our recent animal study demonstrates faster normalization of TRACP-5b levels after discontinuation of RANKL inhibitor OPG-Fc (composed of the RANKL-binding domains of osteoprotegerin linked to the Fc portion of IgG), a surrogate to denosumab, as compared with ZA.[47] In addition, radiographic and histologic indices of ONJ returned to levels of control animals after withdrawal of OPG-Fc, whereas ZA-treated mice still demonstrated ONJ features.[47] If these data can be validated in controlled clinical studies, they may support the rationale for drug holidays in the management of patients with ONJ. They may also demonstrate that discontinuing denosumab versus bisphosphonate therapy before surgical intervention offers faster recovery of normal bone homeostasis.

Another factor that points to the central role of osteoclastic bone resorption in ONJ pathophysiology is the effect of parathyroid hormone (PTH). Initial case reports in osteoporotic patients and animal studies simulating osteoporosis demonstrate the improved healing of extraction sockets and ONJ lesions with administration of PTH, possibly due to its ability to improve bone homeostasis, by directly stimulating osteoblastic function and indirectly increasing osteoclastic bone resorption.[48-51]

Hypothesis 2: Inflammation and Infection

Because only 0.8% to 12.0% of patients on systemic antiresorptives for malignant disease develop ONJ,[3,52-56] although this may be underestimated,[57,58] points to additional inciting factors beside antiresorptives that contribute to ONJ. Valuable information can be gained from patients with ONJ and their coexisting risk factors. Tooth extraction is generally the most common inciting event associated with ONJ, but teeth in adults are almost always extracted because they have periapical or periodontal infections or inflammation.[3,57,59,60] Animal models of inflammation and infection have been developed to parallel the clinical presentation of ONJ with associated dental pathology, and have consistently shown that both inflammation/infection and a systemic antiresorptive are sufficient for ONJ development.[21,33,34,61-65]

Inflammation/infection has been thought to play a role in ONJ, often occurring after extraction of teeth with advanced dental disease or around teeth with periodontal or periapical infection.[3,57,60,66] In patients with multiple myeloma and metastatic cancer, aggressive dental hygiene therapy reduces the incidence of ONJ.[67,68] Further evaluation of histologic specimens detect bacteria on the exposed bone, including *Actinomyces* species.[69,70] However, the question remains: Did the bacteria induce the infection and exposed bone, or did the exposed bone develop a bacterial biofilm? Recent studies have shed light on the complexity of biofilm, which include fungi and viruses in addition to the bacterial species.[71,72] These multiorganism biofilms present challenges to therapy, and may require complicated strategies to eradicate the infection.[73-75]

Hypothesis 3: Angiogenesis Inhibition

Angiogenesis involves the formation of new blood vessels, and necrosis of bones, such as the femur, are usually of vascular etiology.[76] Bone becomes necrotic without adequate blood supply, as do most tissues, even in pathologic processes. Antiangiogenic therapies are now widely used to inhibit tumor invasion and metastases, targeting vascular signaling molecules, such as vascular endothelial growth factor (VEGF).[77] ZA is a known agent that reduces circulating VEGF levels in vivo in patients with cancer and reduces angiogenesis in vitro.[78-80] ZA inhibits proliferation and interferes with adhesion and migration of human endothelial cells,[4,78] which is thought to interrupt tumor invasion and metastases.[4,80] In addition, all BPs, especially nitrogen-containing BPs, induce a statistically significant decrease in microvessel density in vivo.[81]

Recently, new antiangiogenic therapies, such as tyrosine kinase inhibitors and anti-VEGF monoclonal antibodies, are associated with ONJ development.[82-84] For these reasons, the new AAOMS guidelines have recognized antiangiogenics as a contributing factor and modified the disease name to medication-related ONJ (MRONJ).[3] Moreover, the prevalence of ONJ is highest in patients with multiple myeloma, which is thought to be caused by concomitant antiangiogenic medications and steroids.[85,86] Even though there is some evidence that antiangiogenesis is involved in the ONJ disease process, histopathologic studies have shown normal vasculature in postmortem specimens.[36] Most importantly, denosumab has not been associated with antiangiogenesis.[87] Therefore, although unlikely to be central in the development of ONJ, antiangiogenesis is thought to be a significant contributor to the disease process.

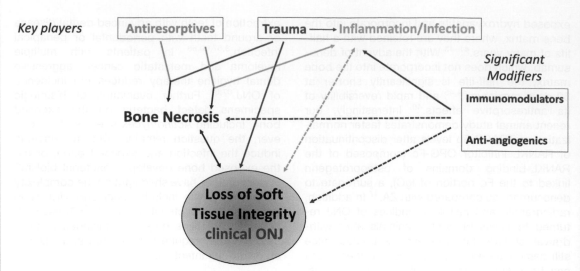

Fig. 1. The potential synergy of multiple pathways of ONJ.

Hypothesis 4: Soft Tissue Toxicity

An early hypothesis in ONJ pathophysiology was a direct soft tissue toxicity of BPs.[88] BP exposure, especially nitrogen-containing BPs, induces apoptosis or decreased proliferation of cervical, prostate, and oral epithelial cells in vitro.[81,88–92] In vitro studies also demonstrate that nitrogen-containing BPs localize to epithelial tissue, as well as bone.[93] In addition, oral alendronate is associated with esophageal irritation, requiring special precautions for patients during administration.[94] However, this hypothesis has become less likely due to the lack of soft tissue toxicity reported with denosumab.

Hypothesis 5: Innate or Acquired Immunity Dysfunction

A continued debate exists about the effect of altered immunity on ONJ development. Tumor pathogenesis is often associated with an impaired immune function,[95] and animal studies have implicated immune deficiency in the development of ONJ, whereas infusion of mesenchymal stem cells or T-regulatory cells prevents and alleviates ONJ-like lesions.[96] In addition, the highest prevalence of ONJ in patients with multiple myeloma, who receive steroids and antiangiogenics as part of their chemotherapy regimen, further points to a role of immune dysfunction in ONJ pathogenesis.[86] Additionally, in many animal models of ONJ, incidence and severity of disease increases with the presence of chemotherapy or steroids.[6,49,63,96,97] In patients on oral BPs, steroids are also a risk factor for ONJ.[3,60] This points to

the potential significant contribution of immunomodulators in the pathophysiology of the disease (**Fig. 1**).

SUMMARY

ONJ is a multifactorial disease in patients with primary or metastatic bone malignancy or osteoporosis undergoing systemic antiresorptive therapy, where the pathophysiology has not yet been fully determined. Human and animal studies point to a combination of mechanisms interacting with each other to increase the development and severity of the disease. The complexity of ONJ and the potential synergy of multiple pathways is depicted on the schematic diagram of **Fig. 1**. Histologic bone necrosis is at the center of the disease process. Strong evidence points to antiresorptives in combination with trauma and/or inflammation/infection as key factors that are necessary and sufficient for ONJ development. Antiresorptives alone do not cause bone necrosis, but when combined with trauma, such as a tooth extraction or inflammation/infection from periodontal or periapical disease, bone necrosis can occur. Necrotic bone in turn can lead to loss of soft tissue integrity, or clinical ONJ. Surgical intervention also results in direct disruption of soft tissues and further complicates the disease. Case reports of exposed, necrotic bone with loss of soft tissue integrity have been associated with trauma or infection alone. Bone exposure propagates infection, and inflammation in a positive feedback loop increases disease severity or extent. Further loss of soft tissue integrity leads to continued bone necrosis, and the cycle perpetuates.

Immunomodulators, such as steroids or chemotherapy, as well as immunocompromised states from disease such as diabetes, and antiangiogenics are significant modifiers that may increase disease prevalence or severity when combined with inflammation/infection or trauma in the presence of antiresorptives. Again, reported cases of ONJ associated with steroids, chemotherapy, or antiangiogenics alone are fewer in number. Bone necrosis does not always lead to bone exposure, which is why stage 0 ONJ has received much attention in recent years. Unless loss of soft tissue integrity occurs, frank bone exposure or stage 1, 2, or 3 clinical ONJ is not diagnosed. Preliminary reports demonstrate that approximately stage 0 ONJ often progresses to clinical bone exposure.[98,99] However, it is unclear what determines progression in those patients. We anticipate that continued preclinical and clinical studies will shed light on the key players and significant modifiers in the development, severity, and progression, and resolution of ONJ. Understanding pathophysiologic mechanisms of ONJ will help explore targeted treatment interventions to reduce development and improve management of patients with established disease.

REFERENCES

1. Khan AA, Morrison A, Hanley DA, et al, International Task Force on Osteonecrosis of the Jaw. Diagnosis and management of osteonecrosis of the jaw: a systematic review and international consensus. J Bone Miner Res 2015;30:3.
2. Ruggiero SL, Dodson TB, Assael LA, et al, American Association of Oral and Maxillofacial Surgeons. American Association of Oral and Maxillofacial Surgeons position paper on bisphosphonate-related osteonecrosis of the jaws–2009 update. J Oral Maxillofac Surg 2009;67:2.
3. Ruggiero SL, Dodson TB, Fantasia J, et al. American Association of Oral and Maxillofacial Surgeons position paper on medication-related osteonecrosis of the jaw–2014 update. J Oral Maxillofac Surg 2014; 72:1938.
4. McLeod NM, Brennan PA, Ruggiero SL. Bisphosphonate osteonecrosis of the jaw: a historical and contemporary review. Surgeon 2012;10:36.
5. Williamson RA. Surgical management of bisphosphonate induced osteonecrosis of the jaws. Int J Oral Maxillofac Surg 2010;39:251.
6. Bi Y, Gao Y, Ehirchiou D, et al. Bisphosphonates cause osteonecrosis of the jaw-like disease in mice. Am J Pathol 2010;177:280.
7. Khosla S, Burr D, Cauley J, et al, American Society for Bone and Mineral Research. Bisphosphonate-associated osteonecrosis of the jaw: report

of a task force of the American Society for Bone and Mineral Research. J Bone Miner Res 2007; 22:1479.
8. Carlson ER, Basile JD. The role of surgical resection in the management of bisphosphonate-related osteonecrosis of the jaws. J Oral Maxillofac Surg 2009;67:85.
9. Carlson ER, Fleisher KE, Ruggiero SL. Metastatic cancer identified in osteonecrosis specimens of the jaws in patients receiving intravenous bisphosphonate medications. J Oral Maxillofac Surg 2013;71(12):2077–86.
10. Spinelli G, Torresetti M, Lazzeri D, et al. Microsurgical reconstruction after bisphosphonate-related osteonecrosis of the jaw: our experience with fibula free flap. J Craniofac Surg 2014;25:788.
11. Marx RE. Pamidronate (Aredia) and zoledronate (Zometa) induced avascular necrosis of the jaws: a growing epidemic. J Oral Maxillofac Surg 2003;61:1115.
12. Ruggiero SL, Mehrotra B, Rosenberg TJ, et al. Osteonecrosis of the jaws associated with the use of bisphosphonates: a review of 63 cases. J Oral Maxillofac Surg 2004;62:527.
13. Baud'huin M, Duplomb L, Ruiz Velasco C, et al. Key roles of the OPG-RANK-RANKL system in bone oncology. Expert Rev Anticancer Ther 2007;7:221.
14. Lacey DL, Boyle WJ, Simonet WS, et al. Bench to bedside: elucidation of the OPG-RANK-RANKL pathway and the development of denosumab. Nat Rev Drug Discov 2012;11:401.
15. Coleman RE, Major P, Lipton A, et al. Predictive value of bone resorption and formation markers in cancer patients with bone metastases receiving the bisphosphonate zoledronic acid. J Clin Oncol 2005;23:4925.
16. Stewart AF. Clinical practice. Hypercalcemia associated with cancer. N Engl J Med 2005; 352:373.
17. Stopeck AT, Lipton A, Body JJ, et al. Denosumab compared with zoledronic acid for the treatment of bone metastases in patients with advanced breast cancer: a randomized, double-blind study. J Clin Oncol 2010;28:5132.
18. Henry DH, Costa L, Goldwasser F, et al. Randomized, double-blind study of denosumab versus zoledronic acid in the treatment of bone metastases in patients with advanced cancer (excluding breast and prostate cancer) or multiple myeloma. J Clin Oncol 2011;29:1125.
19. Allen MR, Burr DB. The pathogenesis of bisphosphonate-related osteonecrosis of the jaw: so many hypotheses, so few data. J Oral Maxillofac Surg 2009;67:61.
20. Rodan GA, Reszka AA. Bisphosphonate mechanism of action. Curr Mol Med 2002;2:571.

21. Aghaloo TL, Kang B, Sung EC, et al. Periodontal disease and bisphosphonates induce osteonecrosis of the jaws in the rat. J Bone Miner Res 2011; 26:1871.

22. Reinwald S, Burr D. Review of nonprimate, large animal models for osteoporosis research. J Bone Miner Res 2008;23:1353.

23. Huja SS, Fernandez SA, Hill KJ, et al. Remodeling dynamics in the alveolar process in skeletally mature dogs. Anat Rec A Discov Mol Cell Evol Biol 2006; 288:1243.

24. Ristow O, Gerngross C, Schwaiger M, et al. Effect of antiresorptive drugs on bony turnover in the jaw: denosumab compared with bisphosphonates. Br J Oral Maxillofac Surg 2014;52:308.

25. Cheong S, Sun S, Kang B, et al. Bisphosphonate uptake in areas of tooth extraction or periapical disease. J Oral Maxillofac Surg 2014;72:2461.

26. Kimmel DB. Mechanism of action, pharmacokinetic and pharmacodynamic profile, and clinical applications of nitrogen-containing bisphosphonates. J Dent Res 2007;86:1022.

27. Baron R, Ferrari S, Russell RG. Denosumab and bisphosphonates: different mechanisms of action and effects. Bone 2011;48:677.

28. Suzuki K, Takeyama S, Sakai Y, et al. Current topics in pharmacological research on bone metabolism: inhibitory effects of bisphosphonates on the differentiation and activity of osteoclasts. J Pharmacol Sci 2006;100:189.

29. Ito M, Amizuka N, Nakajima T, et al. Ultrastructural and cytochemical studies on cell death of osteoclasts induced by bisphosphonate treatment. Bone 1999;25:447.

30. Smith MR, Saad F, Coleman R, et al. Denosumab and bone-metastasis-free survival in men with castration-resistant prostate cancer: results of a phase 3, randomised, placebo-controlled trial. Lancet 2012;379:39.

31. Saad F, Brown JE, Van Poznak C, et al. Incidence, risk factors, and outcomes of osteonecrosis of the jaw: integrated analysis from three blinded active-controlled phase III trials in cancer patients with bone metastases. Ann Oncol 2012;23:1341.

32. Dranitsaris G, Hatzimichael E. Interpreting results from oncology clinical trials: a comparison of denosumab to zoledronic acid for the prevention of skeletal-related events in cancer patients. Support Care Cancer 2012;20:1353.

33. Aghaloo TL, Cheong S, Bezouglaia O, et al. RANK-L inhibitors induce osteonecrosis of the jaw in mice with periapical disease. J Bone Miner Res 2014; 29(4):843–54.

34. Kang B, Cheong S, Chaichanasakul T, et al. Periapical disease and bisphosphonates induce osteonecrosis of the jaws in mice. J Bone Miner Res 2013;28: 1631.

35. Williams DW, Lee C, Kim T, et al. Impaired bone resorption and woven bone formation are associated with development of osteonecrosis of the jaw-like lesions by bisphosphonate and anti-receptor activator of NF-kappaB ligand antibody in mice. Am J Pathol 2014;184:3084.

36. Hellstein JW, Adler RA, Edwards B, et al, American Dental Association Council on Scientific Affairs Expert Panel on Antiresorptive Agents. Managing the care of patients receiving antiresorptive therapy for prevention and treatment of osteoporosis: executive summary of recommendations from the American Dental Association Council on Scientific Affairs. J Am Dent Assoc 2011;142:1243.

37. Woo SB, Hellstein JW, Kalmar JR. Narrative [corrected] review: bisphosphonates and osteonecrosis of the jaws. Ann Intern Med 2006;144:753.

38. Damm DD, Jones DM. Bisphosphonate-related osteonecrosis of the jaws: a potential alternative to drug holidays. Gen Dent 2013;61:33.

39. Lipton A, Fizazi K, Stopeck AT, et al. Superiority of denosumab to zoledronic acid for prevention of skeletal-related events: a combined analysis of 3 pivotal, randomised, phase 3 trials. Eur J Cancer 2012;48:3082.

40. Sinningen K, Tsourdi E, Rauner M, et al. Skeletal and extraskeletal actions of denosumab. Endocrine 2012;42:52.

41. Rogers MJ, Gordon S, Benford HL, et al. Cellular and molecular mechanisms of action of bisphosphonates. Cancer 2000;88:2961.

42. Sato M, Grasser W, Endo N, et al. Bisphosphonate action. Alendronate localization in rat bone and effects on osteoclast ultrastructure. J Clin Invest 1991;88:2095.

43. Shinoda H, Adamek G, Felix R, et al. Structure-activity relationships of various bisphosphonates. Calcif Tissue Int 1983;35:87.

44. Lewiecki EM. Denosumab: an investigational drug for the management of postmenopausal osteoporosis. Biologics 2008;2:645.

45. Lewiecki EM. Denosumab update. Curr Opin Rheumatol 2009;21:369.

46. Silva I, Branco JC. Denosumab: recent update in postmenopausal osteoporosis. Acta Reumatol Port 2012;37:302.

47. de Molon RS, Shimamoto H, Bezouglaia O, et al. OPG-Fc but not zoledronic acid discontinuation reverses osteonecrosis of the jaws (ONJ) in mice. J Bone Miner Res 2015;30(9):1627–40.

48. Kuroshima S, Kovacic BL, Kozloff KM, et al. Intra-oral PTH administration promotes tooth extraction socket healing. J Dent Res 2013;92:553.

49. Kuroshima S, Entezami P, McCauley LK, et al. Early effects of parathyroid hormone on bisphosphonate/steroid-associated compromised osseous wound healing. Osteoporos Int 2014;25:1141.

50. Dayisoylu EH, Senel FC, Ungor C, et al. The effects of adjunctive parathyroid hormone injection on bisphosphonate-related osteonecrosis of the jaws: an animal study. Int J Oral Maxillofac Surg 2013; 42:1475.

51. Duong LT, Rodan GA. Regulation of osteoclast formation and function. Rev Endocr Metab Disord 2001;2:95.

52. Bamias A, Kastritis E, Bamia C, et al. Osteonecrosis of the jaw in cancer after treatment with bisphosphonates: incidence and risk factors. J Clin Oncol 2005;23:8580.

53. Berenson JR, Hillner BE, Kyle RA, et al, American Society of Clinical Oncology Bisphosphonates Expert Panel. American Society of Clinical Oncology clinical practice guidelines: the role of bisphosphonates in multiple myeloma. J Clin Oncol 2002;20:3719.

54. Wang EP, Kaban LB, Strewler GJ, et al. Incidence of osteonecrosis of the jaw in patients with multiple myeloma and breast or prostate cancer on intravenous bisphosphonate therapy. J Oral Maxillofac Surg 2007;65:1328.

55. Zavras AI, Zhu S. Bisphosphonates are associated with increased risk for jaw surgery in medical claims data: is it osteonecrosis? J Oral Maxillofac Surg 2006;64:917.

56. Jadu F, Lee L, Pharoah M, et al. A retrospective study assessing the incidence, risk factors and comorbidities of pamidronate-related necrosis of the jaws in multiple myeloma patients. Ann Oncol 2007;18:2015.

57. Boonyapakorn T, Schirmer I, Reichart PA, et al. Bisphosphonate-induced osteonecrosis of the jaws: prospective study of 80 patients with multiple myeloma and other malignancies. Oral Oncol 2008;44:857.

58. Walter C, Al-Nawas B, Frickhofen N, et al. Prevalence of bisphosphonate associated osteonecrosis of the jaws in multiple myeloma patients. Head Face Med 2010;6:11.

59. Marx R. Oral and intravenous bisphosphonate induced osteonecrosis of the jaws: history, etiology, prevention, and treatment. 2nd edition. Chicago: Quintessence Publishing; 2007.

60. Marx RE, Sawatari Y, Fortin M, et al. Bisphosphonate-induced exposed bone (osteonecrosis/osteopetrosis) of the jaws: risk factors, recognition, prevention, and treatment. J Oral Maxillofac Surg 2005;63:1567.

61. Aguirre JI, Akhter MP, Kimmel DB, et al. Oncologic doses of zoledronic acid induce osteonecrosis of the jaw-like lesions in rice rats (Oryzomys palustris) with periodontitis. J Bone Miner Res 2012;27:2130.

62. Gotcher JE, Jee WS. The progress of the periodontal syndrome in the rice cat. II. The effects of a diphosphonate on the periodontium. J Periodontal Res 1981;16:441.

63. Lopez-Jornet P, Camacho-Alonso F, Martinez-Canovas A, et al. Perioperative antibiotic regimen in rats treated with pamidronate plus dexamethasone and subjected to dental extraction: a study of the changes in the jaws. J Oral Maxillofac Surg 2011;69:2488.

64. Mawardi H, Treister N, Richardson P, et al. Sinus tracts–an early sign of bisphosphonate-associated osteonecrosis of the jaws? J Oral Maxillofac Surg 2009;67:593.

65. de Molon RS, Cheong S, Bezouglaia O, et al. Spontaneous osteonecrosis of the jaws in the maxilla of mice on antiresorptive treatment: a novel ONJ mouse model. Bone 2014;68:11.

66. Ficarra G, Beninati F, Rubino I, et al. Osteonecrosis of the jaws in periodontal patients with a history of bisphosphonates treatment. J Clin Periodontol 2005; 32:1123.

67. Ripamonti CI, Maniezzo M, Campa T, et al. Decreased occurrence of osteonecrosis of the jaw after implementation of dental preventive measures in solid tumour patients with bone metastases treated with bisphosphonates. The experience of the National Cancer Institute of Milan. Ann Oncol 2009;20:137.

68. Dimopoulos MA, Kastritis E, Bamia C, et al. Reduction of osteonecrosis of the jaw (ONJ) after implementation of preventive measures in patients with multiple myeloma treated with zoledronic acid. Ann Oncol 2009;20:117.

69. Hansen T, Kunkel M, Weber A, et al. Osteonecrosis of the jaws in patients treated with bisphosphonates—histomorphologic analysis in comparison with infected osteoradionecrosis. J Oral Pathol Med 2006;35:155.

70. Sedghizadeh PP, Kumar SK, Gorur A, et al. Identification of microbial biofilms in osteonecrosis of the jaws secondary to bisphosphonate therapy. J Oral Maxillofac Surg 2008;66:767.

71. Kumar SK, Gorur A, Schaudinn C, et al. The role of microbial biofilms in osteonecrosis of the jaw associated with bisphosphonate therapy. Curr Osteoporos Rep 2010;8:40.

72. Pushalkar S, Li X, Kurago Z, et al. Oral microbiota and host innate immune response in bisphosphonate-related osteonecrosis of the jaw. Int J Oral Sci 2014; 6:219.

73. Sedghizadeh PP, Kumar SK, Gorur A, et al. Microbial biofilms in osteomyelitis of the jaw and osteonecrosis of the jaw secondary to bisphosphonate therapy. J Am Dent Assoc 2009; 140:1259.

74. Kos M, Junka A, Smutnicka D, et al. Pamidronate enhances bacterial adhesion to bone hydroxyapatite. Another puzzle in the pathology of bisphosphonate-related osteonecrosis of the jaw? J Oral Maxillofac Surg 2013;71:1010.

75. Wanger G, Gorby Y, El-Naggar MY, et al. Electrically conductive bacterial nanowires in bisphosphonate-related osteonecrosis of the jaw biofilms. Oral Surg Oral Med Oral Pathol Oral Radiol 2013;115:71.

76. Zalavras CG, Lieberman JR. Osteonecrosis of the femoral head: evaluation and treatment. J Am Acad Orthop Surg 2014;22:455.

77. Gacche RN, Meshram RJ. Angiogenic factors as potential drug target: efficacy and limitations of anti-angiogenic therapy. Biochim Biophys Acta 2014;161:1846.

78. Wood J, Bonjean K, Ruetz S, et al. Novel antiangiogenic effects of the bisphosphonate compound zoledronic acid. J Pharmacol Exp Ther 2002;302:1055.

79. Bezzi M, Hasmim M, Bieler G, et al. Zoledronate sensitizes endothelial cells to tumor necrosis factor-induced programmed cell death: evidence for the suppression of sustained activation of focal adhesion kinase and protein kinase B/Akt. J Biol Chem 2003;278:43603.

80. Santini D, Vincenzi B, Dicuonzo G, et al. Zoledronic acid induces significant and long-lasting modifications of circulating angiogenic factors in cancer patients. Clin Cancer Res 2003;9:2893.

81. Pabst AM, Ziebart T, Ackermann M, et al. Bisphosphonates' antiangiogenic potency in the development of bisphosphonate-associated osteonecrosis of the jaws: influence on microvessel sprouting in an in vivo 3D Matrigel assay. Clin Oral Investig 2014;18:1015.

82. Guarneri V, Miles D, Robert N, et al. Bevacizumab and osteonecrosis of the jaw: incidence and association with bisphosphonate therapy in three large prospective trials in advanced breast cancer. Breast Cancer Res Treat 2010;122:181.

83. Koch FP, Walter C, Hansen T, et al. Osteonecrosis of the jaw related to sunitinib. Oral Maxillofac Surg 2011;15:63.

84. Santos-Silva AR, Belizario Rosa GA, Castro Junior G, et al. Osteonecrosis of the mandible associated with bevacizumab therapy. Oral Surg Oral Med Oral Pathol Oral Radiol 2013;115:e32.

85. Van den Wyngaert T, Huizing MT, Vermorken JB. Bisphosphonates and osteonecrosis of the jaw: cause and effect or a post hoc fallacy? Ann Oncol 2006;17:1197.

86. Filleul O, Crompot E, Saussez S. Bisphosphonate-induced osteonecrosis of the jaw: a review of 2,400 patient cases. J Cancer Res Clin Oncol 2010;136:1117.

87. Christodoulou C, Pervena A, Klouvas G, et al. Combination of bisphosphonates and antiangiogenic factors induces osteonecrosis of the jaw more frequently than bisphosphonates alone. Oncology 2009;76:209.

88. Reid IR, Bolland MJ, Grey AB. Is bisphosphonate-associated osteonecrosis of the jaw caused by soft tissue toxicity? Bone 2007;41:318.

89. Lin JH. Bisphosphonates: a review of their pharmacokinetic properties. Bone 1996;18:75.

90. Giraudo E, Inoue M, Hanahan D. An amino-bisphosphonate targets MMP-9-expressing macrophages and angiogenesis to impair cervical carcinogenesis. J Clin Invest 2004;114:623.

91. Montague R, Hart CA, George NJ, et al. Differential inhibition of invasion and proliferation by bisphosphonates: anti-metastatic potential of zoledronic acid in prostate cancer. Eur Urol 2004;46:389.

92. Landesberg R, Cozin M, Cremers S, et al. Inhibition of oral mucosal cell wound healing by bisphosphonates. J Oral Maxillofac Surg 2008;66:839.

93. Bae S, Sun S, Aghaloo T, et al. Development of oral osteomucosal tissue constructs in vitro and localization of fluorescently-labeled bisphosphonates to hard and soft tissue. Int J Mol Med 2014;34:559.

94. Watts NB, Diab DL. Long-term use of bisphosphonates in osteoporosis. J Clin Endocrinol Metab 2010;95:1555.

95. Kabilova TO, Kovtonyuk LV, Zonov EV, et al. Immunotherapy of hepatocellular carcinoma with small double-stranded RNA. BMC Cancer 2014;14:338.

96. Kikuiri T, Kim I, Yamaza T, et al. Cell-based immunotherapy with mesenchymal stem cells cures bisphosphonate-related osteonecrosis of the jaw-like disease in mice. J Bone Miner Res 2010;25:1668.

97. Ali-Erdem M, Burak-Cankaya A, Cemil-Isler S, et al. Extraction socket healing in rats treated with bisphosphonate: animal model for bisphosphonate related osteonecrosis of jaws in multiple myeloma patients. Med Oral Patol Oral Cir Bucal 2011;16:e879.

98. Fedele S, Porter SR, D'Aiuto F, et al. Nonexposed variant of bisphosphonate-associated osteonecrosis of the jaw: a case series. Am J Med 2010;123:1060.

99. Patel S, Choyee S, Uyanne J, et al. Non-exposed bisphosphonate-related osteonecrosis of the jaw: a critical assessment of current definition, staging, and treatment guidelines. Oral Dis 2012;18:625.

Medication-Related Osteonecrosis of the Jaw
Basic and Translational Science Updates

Matthew R. Allen, PhD

KEYWORDS

- Bisphosphonates • Denosumab • Antiremodeling agents • ONJ

KEY POINTS

- Basic science advancements in the field of medication-related osteonecrosis of the jaw (MRONJ) have been mainly in our understanding of how agents affect bone and oral epithelial cells.
- A greater understanding exists regarding bisphosphonate accumulation in bone and how this might affect cell function.
- Several animal models, both rodent and large animal, have been developed and have revealed important aspects of MRONJ.
- Basic questions that are essential to our understanding of MRONJ remain unanswered, and having a systemic approach to these questions would accelerate progress of the field.

INTRODUCTION

The clinical description of osteonecrosis of the jaw (ONJ) in 2003–2004,[1,2] along with the increasing reports in the years that followed, caused a significant jolt to those in the field of skeletal biology. Bisphosphonates, a class of antiosteoporotic agents that work by reducing osteoclast activity, were the clinical pillar of excellence in the field.[3] These agents were the most commonly prescribed class of drugs used for treating/preventing osteoporosis,[4] and this efficacy led to their use in numerous other metabolic bone diseases (ie, glucocorticoid-induced osteoporosis) as well as in cancer treatment for reducing skeletal-related events.[5] Significant preclinical and clinical study of bisphosphonates had occurred since the initial work to describe the mechanisms of action[6] and their effects on bone resorption.[7] Yet despite this extensive body of research on bisphosphonates, the clinical description of ONJ (now referred to as MRONJ[8])

made quite apparent the relative paucity of data describing how these agents affect the maxillofacial skeleton.

Over the past decade, progress has been made to understand MRONJ, although in many respects this progress has been faster in the clinical arena than in the basic science arena. It is interesting to think back, just a half dozen years or so, when it was clear that MRONJ was caused by high levels of bisphosphonate accumulation, leading to suppression of intracortical remodeling (which is high in the jaw) and accumulation of large regions of dead/apoptotic osteocytes, which constitute necrotic bone.[9–12] It is now known that nonskeletal accumulating drugs are linked to MRONJ and that MRONJ can be induced in species that do not undergo intracortical remodeling. Yet many questions still remain. The goal of this review is to highlight the key basic science and translational (animal) studies in the area of MRONJ and the needed areas of focus as the field moves forward into the next decade.

Disclosures: The author has no conflicts of interest related to this work.

Department of Anatomy and Cell Biology, Indiana University School of Medicine, 635 Barnhill Drive, MS-5035, Indianapolis, IN 46202, USA

E-mail address: matallen@iupui.edu

Oral Maxillofacial Surg Clin N Am 27 (2015) 497–508
http://dx.doi.org/10.1016/j.coms.2015.06.002

MEDICATION-RELATED OSTEONECROSIS OF THE JAW AT THE CELL LEVEL— BISPHOSPHONATE ACTION ON CELLS AND TISSUE ACCUMULATION

Basic science studies aimed at understanding MRONJ have mainly focused on determining how agents linked to MRONJ affect cell characteristics in vitro. Most of this work has studied bisphosphonates because these were the first, and remain the most common, drug class linked to this condition. Another emerging and exciting area of work, again related to bisphosphonates, is localization of drug within the skeleton.

Years of work, using both in vitro and in vivo model systems, have documented the effects of bisphosphonates on osteoblasts, osteoclasts, and osteocytes.[3] Osteoclast effects depend on the type of bisphosphonate: either by altering ATP metabolism and inducing cell death or by altering the mevalonate pathway that disrupts formation of the small GTPases essential for resorption activity.[13] Osteoclast inhibition, the hallmark of bisphosphonate efficacy, has been confirmed repeatedly in numerous in vitro and in vivo models. Inhibition of osteoclast action seems to clearly be part of the MRONJ pathophysiology, because the agents most commonly linked to MRONJ, bisphosphonates and receptor activator of nuclear factor kappa-B ligand (RANKL) inhibitors (denosumab), both reduce bone resorption, albeit through different mechanisms. Yet the connection to suppression of osteoclasts is not entirely clear because (1) numerous antiresorptive drugs, including estrogen, selective estrogen receptor modulators, and odanacatib, have not been linked to MRONJ and (2) in numerous instances, there are a large number of osteoclasts and/or resorption pits associated with MRONJ lesions.[9,14]

Various hypotheses have been presented regarding these 2 concepts, but definitive data explaining them have yet to be produced.

Necrotic bone is a central component of MRONJ, leading many investigators to focus on the osteocyte. Seminal work aimed at understanding the effects of bisphosphonates on osteocytes has shown that, both in vivo and in vitro, this class of drugs suppresses osteocyte and osteoblast apoptosis.[15] An interesting, and often not appreciated aspect of this work, is that the in vitro studies have repeatedly shown that antiapoptotic effects on osteocytes are dose dependent.[16,17] Although some differences exists among the specific bisphosphonates, concentrations around 10^{-8} M reduced osteocyte apoptosis, whereas those below 10^{-10} M or above 10^{-6} M do not have any effect (Fig. 1). In some instances, the highest doses have levels of apoptosis even above control, potentially suggesting a proapoptotic action at very high doses (above 10^{-5} M). Imaging studies have clearly shown that bisphosphonates can reach osteocyte lacunae,[18,19] yet the concentrations to which these cells are exposed in vivo remain unknown. Given the antiapoptotic effect observed in vivo,[15] it is assumed that they reach levels around 10^{-8} M, but neither has this been confirmed nor is it known whether it is possible, with prolonged or high-dose treatment, to achieve toxic doses.

In vitro assessment of other cells, specifically those of the oral cavity (oral epithelial cells [keratinocytes] and fibroblasts), has increased in the recent literature because of the potential relevance of soft tissue toxicity in MRONJ. In most cases, these studies have revealed that bisphosphonates reduce cell proliferation, induce apoptosis, and slow cell migration (as examples, see[20–23]). These studies typically involve using either primary cells

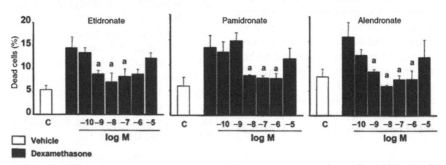

Fig. 1. Effects of bisphosphonates on osteocyte apoptosis are concentration dependent. Using an MLO-Y4 osteocytic cell apoptosis model, the ability of various concentrations of several bisphophonates to inhibit dexamethasone-induced cell death was assessed. The results show that at concentrations between 10^{-9} M and 10^{-6} M bisphophonates effectively prevent dexamethasone-induced apoptosis. Interestingly, at higher concentrations, the effect is lost and apoptosis is no different from that in untreated controls. [a] P<.05 versus dexamethasone treatment alone. (*Adapted from* Plotkin L, Weinstein R, Parfitt A, et al. Prevention of osteocyte and osteoblast apoptosis by bisphosphonates and calcitonin. J Clin Invest 1999;104(10):1363–74; with permission.)

from animals/humans or cell lines and then exposing the cells to various bisphosphonates. Although such studies yield important data, they are limited by the fact that it remains unclear if cells of the oral cavity would be exposed to sufficiently high concentrations of bisphosphonate to induce these effects. Concentrations to which osteocytes might be exposed are not known, and there is even less understanding about how bisphosphonates that are within the bone might (or might not) be liberated into the local environment to influence adjacent cells of the oral mucosa.

Using a creative experimental setup, epithelial cells (colorectal adenocarcinoma and ovarian cell lines) were cultured on bone slices that were presoaked with bisphosphonate (or control) to determine the effects of bound drug (as opposed to experimental setups in which the drug is added to the media).[24] The investigators showed that cells adhered to the bone slices similarly in both experimental conditions. Over time, cell proliferation occurred in control conditions, whereas it did not occur on bisphosphonate-soaked slices (**Fig. 2**). These effects depended on the concentration of bisphosphonate that the bone was soaked in (only occurring at concentrations >10 μM), although there was no assessment of actual amounts of drug on the bone surface. In addition,

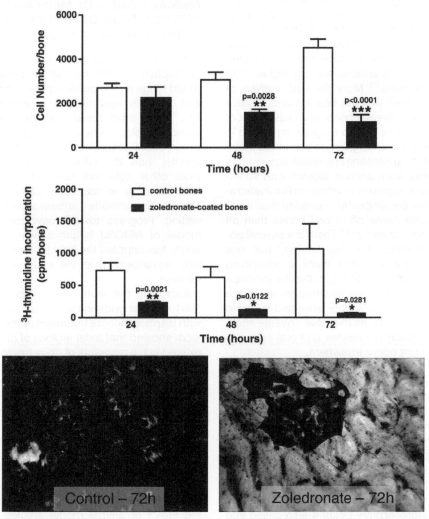

Fig. 2. Alterations in epithelial cells grown on bisphosphonate-soaked bone matrix. In an attempt to mimic what epithelial cells would experience in vivo, bone matrix was presoaked in zoledronic acid (or control) and then cells were seeded to assess growth and proliferation (thymidine incorporation). Superscript letters denote significant differences from control at each time point: [a] P<0.05; [b] P<0.01; [c] P<0.0001; n = 6 in each group. The lower panel shows typical cultures at 72 hours, with the zoledronate-treated bones having substantial areas that were free of cells. (*From* Cornish J, Bava U, Callon KE, et al. Bone-bound bisphosphonate inhibits growth of adjacent non-bone cells. Bone 2011;49(4):710–6; with permission.)

the investigators found differences in the magnitude of effect among the various bisphosphonates (greatest inhibition by zoledronate, ibandronate, and alendronate). These types of experiments, using bone from animals or patients exposed to bisphosphonates, could provide great insight into understanding how bisphosphonates might be affecting nearby oral mucosa cells.

Skeletal accumulation of bisphosphonates has long been hypothesized to play a role in MRONJ despite little data concerning accumulation.[9,25] The development of fluorescent-tagged compounds has allowed questions to be answered that could previously be addressed only using radiolabeled compounds.[26] Comparative studies suggest that higher amounts of labeled bisphosphonate are taken up in the mandible of rats than in the femur, although the difference was modest (about 20% higher in the mandible than in the femur).[27] Other studies have suggested that levels in the mandible are not higher than those in other sites.[28] More detailed analysis of localization showed that bisphosphonates localize in the molar root, alveolar bone, and incisor root of rats (Fig. 3).[29] There is also drug accumulation in the teeth (dentin-enamel junction and in the molar dentin space).[29] Interesting and novel experiments in which bones from animals labeled with florescent drug were exposed to ethylenediaminetetraacetic acid for decalcification revealed that more bisphosphonate came off of oral bones than off the appendicular skeleton.[28] There are several potential explanations for this finding, but one intriguing possibility is that there is something unique about the drug binding in the jaw (perhaps differences in the mineral structure to which the drug binds) that makes it more labile and by doing so, allows concentrations that have adverse effect on local cells (both osteocytes and oral epithelial cells) that do not occur elsewhere.

Following years of belief that jaw necrosis was a complication limited to bisphosphonate treatment, reports of similar jaw necrosis in patients treated with denosumab,[30–32] an inhibitor of the RANKL/RANK signaling pathway of osteoclast development, provided convincing evidence that potent suppression of osteoclasts was part of the pathophysiology. This knowledge resulted in a transition to the idea of jaw necrosis being linked to antiresorptive agents (and the terminology change to antiresorptive ONJ); it also called into question the importance of drug accumulation as part of the pathophysiology. At this point, although high accumulation of drug seems unlikely to be a major driver of the pathophysiology, it may still have a role and probably deserves continued exploration.

Most recently, antiangiogenic medications and inhibitors of vascular endothelial growth factors have each been linked to jaw necrosis (hence yet another terminology change, this time to MRONJ). These drugs have been linked mostly in the form of case reports[33] with larger cohort studies failing to show independent effects.[34] The effects of anti-RANKL agents, antiangiogenic medications, and vascular endothelial growth factors on osteocyte viability or oral epithelial cells necessitate further study and should be a focus in the coming years to understand what commonalities exist between these and bisphosphonates and thus might represent a common pathophysiology mechanism.

ANIMAL MODELS OF MEDICATION-RELATED OSTEONECROSIS OF THE JAW: THE TOOLBOX IS FULL AND READY TO BE PUT TO WORK

It was clear from the early days after the clinical description of MRONJ that significant progress would hinge on the development of animal models that faithfully replicated the clinical manifestation.[35] The most basic questions regarding the pathophysiology, such as what was the exact cause/effect of bisphosphonates (and now other agents), how dose/duration played a role, and what other cofactors were major contributors, were possible to assess in clinical studies but could be expeditiously answered in the preclinical setting. Progress toward developing an animal model of MRONJ began slowly, and in many ways, this crippled the field for several years with little advancement in the understanding of the disease.

Excluding the work of Gotcher and Jee[36] in 1981, the first evidence of jaw necrosis associated with bisphosphonate treatment came in 2008. This work showed that focal regions of nonviable bone existed in the mandible of dogs treated for 3 years with bisphosphonates (but was completely absent in control animals).[37] Although intriguing to consider the link to MRONJ, the absence of exposed bone made it unclear how applicable these findings were to the clinical condition. After 1 year, perhaps one of the most highly influential MRONJ animal model article was published, which showed exposed bone in rats following the combination of dental surgery, bisphosphonates, and dexamethasone.[38] This finding set off a domino effect of animal model articles, which now number over 4 dozen, describing how various combinations of interventions are (or are not) associated with MRONJ-related criteria (see tables in recent reviews[39,40]). Although beneficial, as this work has illustrated the strengths/weaknesses of various models, in some ways, the energy put

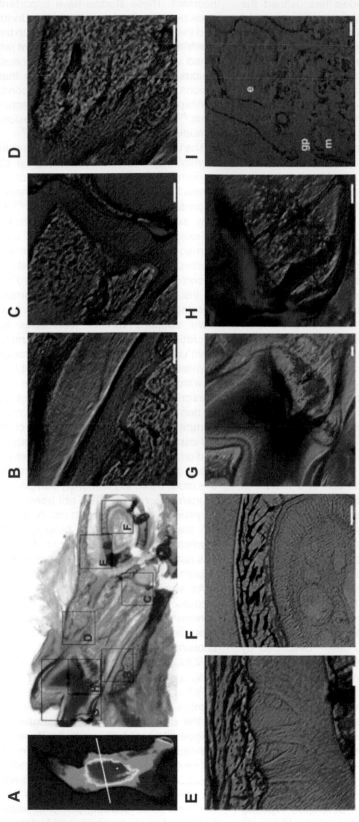

Fig. 3. Localization of bisphosphonate in the mandible. In situ fluorescence of far-red fluorescent pamidronate (FRFP) signal (*red*) in the mandible demonstrates widespread bisphosphonate localization. (*A*) The 2.5× overview highlighting locations of subsequent 10× (*G*) and 20× panels (*B–F, H*). (Inset) Whole-mandible fluorescence and location of frontal section. (*B*) Alveolar bone adjacent to periodontal ligament. (*C*) Base of molar root. (*D*) Alveolar bone. (*E*) Bone surrounding incisor-periodontal ligament space. (*F*) Incisor dentin-enamel junction. (*G*) ×10 magnification of molar dentin space. (*H*) ×20 magnification of panel G showing molar dentin space and supplying vasculature. (*I*) Fluorescence FRFP signal in the proximal femur shows FRFP binding in the epiphyseal (e) and metaphyseal (m) regions. Growth plate (gp) is shown for reference. Scale bar = 50 μm. (*From* Kozloff KM, Volakis LI, Marini JC, Marini JC, et al. Near-infrared fluorescent probe traces bisphosphonate delivery and retention in vivo. J Bone Miner Res 2010;25(8):1748–58; with permission.)

into developing animal models has defined the field, as opposed to using animal models to answer questions about the pathophysiology.

Animal model development has been predominantly undertaken in rodents (rats and mice). Although rodents have numerous advantages as a research model, most notably the ability for genetic manipulation, one limitation from a skeletal physiology standpoint is the lack of remodeling within cortical bone (called osteonal or intracortical remodeling)[41] in the absence of interventions (such as estrogen withdrawal, calcium restriction, induction of microdamage).[42,43] Given that most early evidence suggested remodeling suppression is a key component of MRONJ, and the human mandible has high rates of intracortical remodeling, the applicability of rodent bone was questioned,[35] leading to several studies using large animal models (dogs and pigs) that have cortical bone physiology more similar to humans.[44] Nonetheless, repeated studies have shown that MRONJ can be induced in rats/mice, raising the question of whether intracortical remodeling suppression is really part of the pathophysiology.

Rodent Models

The first animal model to document clinical manifestations of MRONJ was published by Sonis and colleagues[38] and showed visual and radiographic effects consistent with clinical disease. Using young, growing rats, treated with a combination of zoledronic acid and dexamethasone and then subjected to extraction of 3 molars in the mandible or maxilla, mucosal ulceration developed and persisted in experimental animals to a greater degree than controls. Since the work of Sonis and colleagues,[38] dozens of similar studies have been published describing how bisphosphonates, with or without dental perturbation or coadministration of other drugs, lead to the manifestation (or lack) of ONJ in rats and mice. Some of the more intriguing and informative of these studies are discussed below.

The work of Gotcher and Jee,[36] described by some as the first model of MRONJ, used a special strain of rat (the marsh rice rat) that was susceptible to periodontitis when fed soft food. Revisiting this rat strain has shown that these animals develop prominent periodontal lesions but only zoledronate-treated animals develop exposed bone (**Fig. 4**). Similar results have been shown in Sprague Dawley rats induced to have periodontitis using a common ligature model.[45] In the ligature model, animals with periodontal disease and treated with bisphosphonate developed exposed bone, sequestra formation, and histologic

necrosis. These studies have important implications because they show that periodontal disease and the local changes associated with this disease (such as inflammation) are sufficient when combined with bisphosphonates to manifest MRONJ lesions. Other models have shown that MRONJ lesions can be produced when combining bisphosphonates with localized bacterial injections,[46] induction of periapical lesions,[47,48] or denuding the palatal bone gingiva.[49]

The far more common approach in animal model development, driven by the clinical data, is to perform dental extractions in bisphosphonate-treated animals. Dozens of studies have used this approach with variable outcomes.[39,40] It is unclear why such study variability in outcome exists, although in some cases the types of assessments carried out have varied considerably across studies. The easiest and most consistent outcome to compare across studies is exposed bone based on visual examination. Other outcomes, such as histologic necrosis, are more vague. Investigators have adopted various techniques to identify necrotic tissue, including regions of matrix lacking stain uptake (indicating nonpatent canaliculi) and nonviable osteocytes, and also variable definitions of what constitutes nonviable tissue (some using area criteria and other using a threshold for number of nonviable osteocytes). Another challenge for comparing across studies is the use of different bisphosphonates, different routes of administration, and different doses/dosing scheduled. Any or all of these could affect the results, and unfortunately, the most basic experiments, comparing different drugs/routes/doses, have not been undertaken in a systematic way. This fact has hindered the field by leading to extreme heterogeneity among studies and, from a translational point of view, has not informed clinicians on the most important aspects of dosing to reduce the risk of MRONJ.

As significant as the work of Sonis and colleagues[38] was in showing a link between bisphosphonates and MRONJ in an animal model was the work of Aghaloo and colleagues[50] in showing a link between RANKL inhibitors and MRONJ.[51] Denosumab, the only other antiremodeling agent that has shown clinical manifestation of MRONJ,[31] is important to MRONJ because it represents a second antiremodeling treatment linked to the disease. In their work, Aghaloo and colleagues[50] treated mice with 2 different analogs of denosumab, receptor activator of nuclear factor kappa-B immunoglobulin Fc segment complex (RANK-Fc) or osteoprotegerin- immunoglobulin Fc segment complex (OPG-Fc) and found exposed bone following pulpal exposure in 20% to 30% of treated animals and histologic necrosis

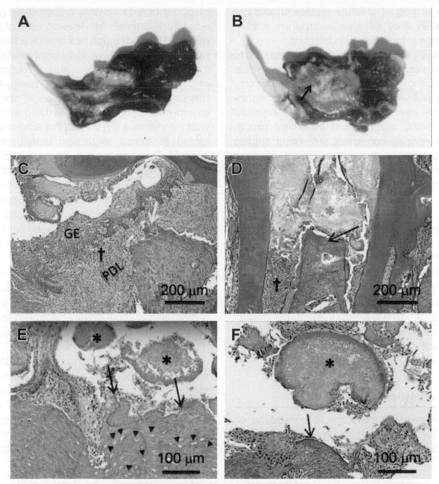

Fig. 4. Example of a rodent model of MRONJ. MRONJ-like lesions observed in mandibles from male rice rats treated with vehicle (*A*) or a high dose (80 mg/kg) of zoledronate (*B*) for 24 weeks. ONJ-like lesions are grossly characterized by extensive ulceration of the gingiva (*arrow*), exposed alveolar bone, molar furcation, and loss of tooth support. Histologic images of mandibles (except in D, which is from maxilla) from female rice rats treated with vehicle (*C*) and high-dose zoledronate (HD-ZOL) for 24 weeks (*D–F*). Photos were taken at the interproximal space between the first and second molars. Several vehicle-treated rats developed severe periodontitis after 24 weeks of treatment in C. Note the substantial hyperplasia of the gingival epithelium (GE), inflammatory cell infiltration of the lamina propria (*), disruption of the periodontal ligament (PDL), apical migration of the junctional epithelium (green arrowhead), and alveolar bone crest resorption (*yellow arrow*). Only rats treated with HD-ZOL develop MRONJ-like lesions. These lesions are characterized by the presence of exposed necrotic alveolar bone (*black arrows*) in D–F, severe inflammatory cell infiltrate (*), and bacterial biofilm morphologically resembling *Actinomyces* sp (*black asterisks*). Note the substantial disruption of the periodontium, ulceration of the gingival epithelium, massive accumulation of bacterial plaque (*green asterisk*), exposed necrotic alveolar bone (*black arrow*) in the maxilla of a rat treated with HD-ZOL for 24 weeks in D. *Actinomyces*-like colonies (*asterisks*) are found attached to necrotic alveolar bone in D–F, or on the surface of ulcerated periodontium adjacent to soft tissue or bone in E and F. A classic sulfur granule of *Actinomyces*-like organism is observed in the interproximal space (*asterisk*). Necrotic alveolar bone was characterized histologically by extensive areas with empty osteocyte lacunae (*black arrowheads*) in E. (*C, D*) Hematoxylin-eosin, bars = 200 μm; (*E, F*) hematoxylin-eosin, bars = 100 μm. (*From* Aguirre JI, Akhter MP, Kimmel DB, et al. Oncologic doses of zoledronic acid induce osteonecrosis of the jaw-like lesions in rice rats [*Oryzomys palustris*] with periodontitis. J Bone Miner Res 2012;27(10):2130–43; with permission.)

in all animals. Follow-up studies showed that even in the absence of periodontal disease, mice treated with zoledronic acid, RANK-Fc, or OPG-Fc that naturally develop oral infection developed exposed bone.[51] Combining anti-RANKL with dental extraction also produces exposed bone in mice at rates comparable to those produced by bisphosphonates.[52] These later studies, controlled experiments comparing/contrasting bisphosphonates and RANKL inhibition, serve as a template regarding what future studies should undertake. Ideally they will also incorporate antiangiogenic drugs into these comparisons.

Animal studies have not been undertaken to study how antiangiogenic drugs may play a role in MRONJ pathology, yet recent data have combined chemotherapeutics with bisphosphonates.[53] The investigators observed exposed bone only in the combination treatment group, which is not entirely consistent with other studies in which bisphosphonates were sufficient to induce exposed bone. However, the most interesting and novel observation from this experiment was the quantification of alterations in lymphatic vessels. Specifically, necrotic lesions had less numbers of lymphatic vessels and less signaling molecules for lymphangiogenesis. Similar, but less-dramatic, effects were shown in animals treated with a combination of bisphosphonates and chemotherapeutics that did not develop necrotic bone. As bisphosphonate treatment alone did not result in changes to the lymph system, the degree to which these changes are relevant to MRONJ is not clear, but the results are intriguing enough that further work should be undertaken in this area.

Large Animal Models

Given the presence of intracortical remodeling, as well as the early data describing necrotic bone in the oral cavity of dogs following long-term bisphosphonate treatment,[37] multiple groups pursued large animals for development of an MRONJ model. Although much has been learned in the dog model, regarding how bisphosphonates affect intracortical remodeling and extraction healing,[14,54–57] overt MRONJ (as clinically defined) has only been reported in a single animal. In that experiment (lasting for 3 months) 1 animal treated with intravenous (IV) zoledronic acid and then subjected to dental extraction developed exposed bone.[14] This exposed bone matched several of the clinical criteria for ONJ including the production of a sequestrum. Follow-up experiments, in which animals were treated for longer durations with IV zoledronic acid before dental extraction, failed to produce exposed bone in any animal, even in those animals in which zoledronic acid was combined with dexamethasone (a common cofactor in clinical MRONJ).[54] Collectively, studies in the dog model have shown that bisphosphonates produce a clear suppression of intracortical remodeling and negatively affect osseous healing. However, the model does not produce a robust manifestation of exposed bone.

The other large animal species investigated as a model of MRONJ is the swine. Using skeletally mature mini pigs, bisphosphonate treatment combined with dental extraction resulted in exposed bone in all animals (**Fig. 5**).[58] This study could be considered a gold standard for preclinical assessment of an animal model, because it conducted a

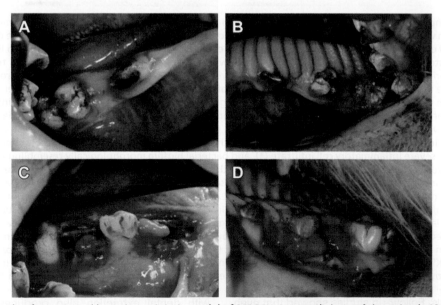

Fig. 5. Example of an exposed bone in a mini pig model of MRONJ. Intraoral views of the animals 10 weeks after teeth extractions with uneventful wound healing in the control group ([A] mandible; [B] maxilla). In contrast, all animals in the bisphosphonate group showed impaired healing and exposed bone ([C] mandible; [D] maxilla). (*From* Pautke C, Kreutzer K, Weitz J, et al. Bisphosphonate related osteonecrosis of the jaw: A minipig large animal model. Bone 2012;51:1–34; with permission.)

robust analysis of several factors related to necrosis—effectively showing visual, histologic, and computed-tomographic-based evidence of MRONJ. Unfortunately, this study neither measured intracortical bone turnover rates nor commented on the amount of osteonal bone within the mandible tissue of mini pigs. A second mini pig study, again using a combination of bisphosphonate and dental extraction, showed exposed bone.[59] Most excitingly, this latter study was able to rescue the exposed bone using mesenchymal stem cell therapy.

WHERE DO WE GO FROM HERE?

The field has made great strides in understanding MRONJ, not only from basic/translational studies but also from significant clinical work (expertly reviewed in other articles of this special issue). Much more is known now than 10 years ago when MRONJ was first described clinically including a basic understanding of the connection between drugs that potentially suppress remodeling and jaw necrosis. There are also several animal models in which to study focused questions. Potential therapies, with some level of success, are already being tested in both small and large animal models.[59,60] These interventional studies are great, and will help provide critical data needed to evaluate potential therapies. But the fact that some of the most basic studies related to MRONJ have not been conducted should not be ignored.

No studies to date have systematically compared, in a model in which exposed bone manifests, the different bisphosphonates to understand if there are truly differences, when variables such as dose and route of administration are matched. Similarly, studies in which dose and duration (which in some ways are linked but can be experimentally decoupled) are independently assessed to determine if either predominates in the manifestation of disease are lacking. These simple questions that are sometimes viewed as nonmechanistic and therefore of low scientific rigor are absolutely essential to the understanding of the disease. It is unfortunate that they have not been addressed in the past 10 years.

One challenge in answering these questions is in determining, for an individual study, which of the many animal models to use. The rodent models seem most robust, and given the ease of access for most investigators, and the relatively low cost, these likely represent the initial models of choice. Yet because of the fundamental differences in remodeling of cortical bone between rodents and larger species, and the exciting emergence of the swine model (and to a lesser degree the dog model), those findings that seem to be most promising from rodents should be confirmed in a larger animal model.

An interesting finding that has emerged in several articles from across all animal models (mice, rats, dogs, swine) and in human imaging studies is new periosteal bone formation (**Fig. 6**). This bone can be observed in control animals but is most prominent in animals treated with antiresorptive agents (both bisphosphonates and RANK inhibitors). This observation has also been documented in several clinical MRONJ articles. The reason for this new bone formation is not clear, but it is an area that is apt for exploration because it could represent a marker of MRONJ that could be imaged noninvasively (if it exists before bone exposure).

It also remains unclear if the various agents linked to MRONJ all work through a common mechanism. Although it seems unlikely that multiple mechanisms would exist, it remains possible and needs to be ruled out as best possible. In the same way, it is unclear how drug holidays, an emerging concept related to reducing the risk of MRONJ,[61] affect the risk of this condition. Studies of drug holidays could easily be undertaken in an animal model and would have important translational value. There are also emerging clinical reports of various treatment modalities for existing MRONJ (such as parathyroid hormone [PTH][62]). These promising treatments can and should be tested rigorously in preclinical models.

Finally, it would seem beneficial to develop a more systematic approach to studying MRONJ among interested investigators. Science is inherently competitive with those on the cutting edge of discovery reaping benefits through both funding and advancement. Yet it is a matter of consideration as to where we might be if a more coordinated approach to developing an animal model had been taken from the outset. Rather than dozens of individual laboratory-conducive experiments, that are similar in many respects but not enough to directly compare, this effort could have been mapped out in a divide-and-conquer approach. Models could have been developed and replicated in a fraction of time. What has been done is done, but the field now has yet another opportunity to approach the relevant basic science issues related to MRONJ. Brining together parties that are interested in working as a group to advance our basic science understanding of this condition could galvanize the field into action. Most importantly, it could produce a roadmap that clearly outlines not only the destination but also the road to get there in order to assure that in another decade we can look back and declare a more complete understanding of MRONJ.

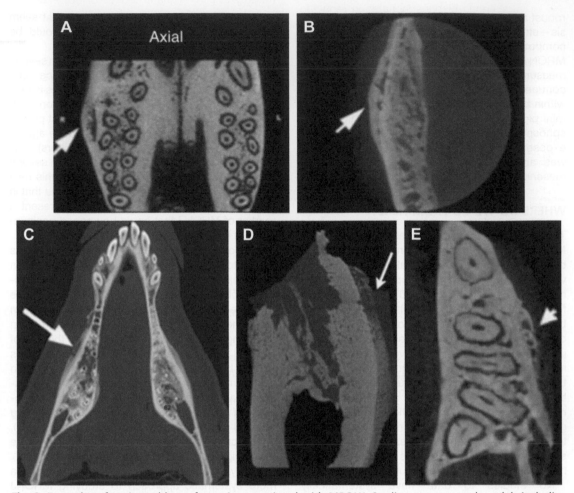

Fig. 6. Examples of periosteal bone formation associated with MRONJ. Studies across several models including rats (*A*), humans (*B*), mini pigs (*C*), dogs (*D*), and mice (*E*) have revealed such formation (*arrows*), yet little is known about its role in MRONJ pathophysiology or if it could be used an imaging marker. (*From* Allen MR. Animal models of medication-related osteonecrosis of the jaw. In: Otto S. *Editor*. Medication-related osteonecrosis of the jaws. Berlin: Springer Berlin Heidelberg; 2014. p. 155–67; with permission.)

REFERENCES

1. Ruggiero SL, Mehrotra B, Rosenberg TJ, et al. Osteonecrosis of the jaws associated with the use of bisphosphonates: a review of 63 cases. J Oral Maxillofac Surg 2004;62(5):527–34.
2. Marx R. Pamidronate (Aredia) and zoledronate (Zometa) induced avascular necrosis of the jaws: a growing epidemic. J Oral Maxillofac Surg 2003; 61(9):1115.
3. Russell RG. Bisphosphonates: the first 40 years. Bone 2011;49(1):2–19.
4. Eastell R, Walsh JS, Watts NB, et al. Bisphosphonates for postmenopausal osteoporosis. Bone 2011;49(1):82–8.
5. Coleman RE, McCloskey EV. Bisphosphonates in oncology. Bone 2011;49(1):71–6.
6. Francis M, Graham R, Russell G, et al. Diphosphonates inhibit formation of calcium phosphate crystals in vitro and pathological calcification in vivo. Science 1969;165(3899):1264.
7. Schenk R, Merz W, Mühlbauer R, et al. Effect of ethane-1-hydroxy-1, 1-diphosphonate (EHDP) and dichloromethylene diphosphonate (Cl 2 MDP) on the calcification and resorption of cartilage and bone in the tibial epiphysis and metaphysis of rats. Calcif Tissue Int 1973;11(3):196–214.
8. Ruggiero SL, Dodson TB, Fantasia J, et al. American Association of Oral and Maxillofacial Surgeons position paper on medication-related osteonecrosis of the jaw-2014 update. J Oral Maxillofac Surg 2014; 72(10):1938–56.
9. Allen MR, Burr DB. The pathogenesis of bisphosphonate-related osteonecrosis of the jaw:

so many hypotheses, so few data. J Oral Maxillofac Surg 2009;67(5):61–70.

10. Woo SB, Hellstein JW, Kalmar JR. Systematic review: bisphosphonates and osteonecrosis of the jaws. Ann Intern Med 2006;144:753–61.

11. Reid IR, Bolland MJ, Grey AB. Is bisphosphonate-associated osteonecrosis of the jaw caused by soft tissue toxicity? Bone 2007;41(3):318–20.

12. Somerman MJ, McCauley LK. Bisphosphonates: sacrificing the jaw to save the skeleton? International Bone and Mineral Society Knowledge Environment 2006;3(9):12–8.

13. Rogers MJ, Crockett JC, Coxon FP, et al. Biochemical and molecular mechanisms of action of bisphosphonates. Bone 2011;49(1):34–41.

14. Allen MR, Kubek DJ, Burr DB, et al. Compromised osseous healing of dental extraction sites in zoledronic acid-treated dogs. Osteoporos Int 2011; 22(2):693–702.

15. Bellido T, Plotkin LI. Novel actions of bisphosphonates in bone: preservation of osteoblast and osteocyte viability. Bone 2011;49(1):50–5.

16. Plotkin L, Weinstein R, Parfitt A, et al. Prevention of osteocyte and osteoblast apoptosis by bisphosphonates and calcitonin. J Clin Invest 1999;104(10): 1363–74.

17. Plotkin L, Manolagas S, Bellido T. Dissociation of the pro-apoptotic effects of bisphosphonates on osteoclasts from their anti-apoptotic effects on osteoblasts/osteocytes with novel analogs. Bone 2006; 39(3):443–52.

18. Turek J, Ebetino FH, Lundy MW, et al. Bisphosphonate binding affinity affects drug distribution in both intracortical and trabecular bone of rabbits. Calcif Tissue Int 2012;90(3):202–10.

19. Roelofs AJ, Coxon FP, Ebetino FH, et al. Fluorescent risedronate analogues reveal bisphosphonate uptake by bone marrow monocytes and localization around osteocytes in vivo. J Bone Miner Res 2010; 25(3):606–16.

20. Landesberg R, Cozin M, Cremers S, et al. Inhibition of oral mucosal cell wound healing by bisphosphonates. J Oral Maxillofac Surg 2008; 66(5):839–47.

21. Landesberg R, Woo V, Cremers S, et al. Potential pathophysiological mechanisms in osteonecrosis of the jaw. Ann N Y Acad Sci 2011;1218(1):62–79.

22. Ravosa MJ, Ning J, Liu Y, et al. Bisphosphonate effects on the behaviour of oral epithelial cells and oral fibroblasts. Arch Oral Biol 2011;56(5):491–8.

23. Pabst AM, Ziebart T, Koch FP, et al. The influence of bisphosphonates on viability, migration, and apoptosis of human oral keratinocytes—in vitro study. Clin Oral Investig 2011;16(1):87–93.

24. Cornish J, Bava U, Callon KE, et al. Bone-bound bisphosphonate inhibits growth of adjacent non-bone cells. Bone 2011;49(4):710–6.

25. Allen MR. Skeletal accumulation of bisphosphonates: implications for osteoporosis treatment. Expert Opin Drug Metab Toxicol 2008;4(11):1371–8.

26. Sato M, Grasser W, Endo N, et al. Bisphosphonate action. Alendronate localization in rat bone and effects on osteoclast ultrastructure. J Clin Invest 1991;88(6):2095.

27. Hokugo A, Sun S, Park S, et al. Equilibrium-dependent bisphosphonate interaction with crystalline bone mineral explains anti-resorptive pharmacokinetics and prevalence of osteonecrosis of the jaw in rats. Bone 2013;53(1):59–68.

28. Wen D, Qing L, Harrison G, et al. Anatomic site variability in rat skeletal uptake and desorption of fluorescently labeled bisphosphonate. Oral Dis 2011; 17(4):427–32.

29. Kozloff KM, Volakis LI, Marini JC, et al. Near-infrared fluorescent probe traces bisphosphonate delivery and retention in vivo. J Bone Miner Res 2010; 25(8):1748–58.

30. Taylor K, Middlefell L, Mizen K. Osteonecrosis of the jaws induced by anti-RANK ligand therapy. Br J Oral Maxillofac Surg 2010;48(3):221–3.

31. Aghaloo TL, Felsenfeld AL, Tetradis S. Osteonecrosis of the jaw in a patient on Denosumab. J Oral Maxillofac Surg 2010;68(5):959–63.

32. Kyrgidis A, Toulis K. Denosumab-related osteonecrosis of the jaws. Osteoporos Int 2010;22:1–2.

33. Estilo CL, Fornier M, Farooki A, et al. Osteonecrosis of the jaw related to bevacizumab. J Clin Oncol 2008;26(24):4037–8.

34. Guarneri V, Miles D, Robert N, et al. Bevacizumab and osteonecrosis of the jaw: incidence and association with bisphosphonate therapy in three large prospective trials in advanced breast cancer. Breast Cancer Res Treat 2010;122(1):181–8.

35. Allen MR. Animal models of osteonecrosis of the jaw. J Musculoskelet Neuronal Interact 2007;7(4): 358–60.

36. Gotcher J, Jee W. The progress of the periodontal syndrome in the rice rat. J Periodont Res 1981; 16(3):275–91.

37. Allen MR, Burr DB. Mandible matrix necrosis in beagle dogs after 3 years of daily oral bisphosphonate treatment. J Oral Maxillofac Surg 2008;66(5): 987–94.

38. Sonis ST, Watkins BA, Lyng GD, et al. Bony changes in the jaws of rats treated with zoledronic acid and dexamethasone before dental extractions mimic bisphosphonate-related osteonecrosis in cancer patients. Oral Oncol 2009;45(2):164–72.

39. Allen MR. Animal models of medication-related osteonecrosis of the jaw. In: Otto S, editor. Medication-related osteonecrosis of the jaws. Berlin: Springer Berlin Heidelberg; 2014. p. 155–67.

40. Allen MR, Ruggiero SL. A review of pharmaceutical agents and oral bone health: how osteonecrosis of

the jaw has affected the field. Int J Oral Maxillofac Implants 2014;29(1):e45–57.

41. Jowsey J. Studies of Haversian systems in man and some animals. J Anat 1966;100(Pt 4):857–64.

42. Kubek D, Burr D, Allen M. Ovariectomy stimulates and bisphosphonates inhibit intracortical remodeling in the mouse mandible. Orthod Craniofac Res 2010;13(4):214–22.

43. Bentolila V, Boyce T, Fyhrie D, et al. Intracortical remodeling in adult rat long bones after fatigue loading. Bone 1998;23(3):275–81.

44. Reinwald S, Burr D. Review of nonprimate, large animal models for osteoporosis research. J Bone Miner Res 2008;23(9):1353–68.

45. Aghaloo TL, Kang B, Sung EC, et al. Periodontal disease and bisphosphonates induce osteonecrosis of the jaws in the rat. J Bone Miner Res 2011;26(8): 1871–82.

46. Tsurushima H, Kokuryo S, Sakaguchi O, et al. Bacterial promotion of bisphosphonate-induced osteonecrosis in Wistar rats. Int J Oral Maxillofac Surg 2013;42(11):1481–7.

47. Kang B, Cheong S, Chaichanasakul T, et al. Periapical disease and bisphosphonates induce osteonecrosis of the jaws in mice. J Bone Miner Res 2013; 28(7):1631–40.

48. Xiong H, Wei L, Hu Y, et al. Effect of alendronate on alveolar bone resorption and angiogenesis in rats with experimental periapical lesions. Int Endod J 2010;43(6):485–91.

49. Yamashita J, Koi K, Yang D-Y, et al. Effect of zoledronate on oral wound healing in rats. Clin Cancer Res 2011;17(6):1405–14.

50. Aghaloo TL, Cheong S, Bezouglaia O, et al. RANKL inhibitors induce osteonecrosis of the jaw in mice with periapical disease. J Bone Miner Res 2014; 29(4):843–54.

51. de Molon RS, Cheong S, Bezouglaia O, et al. Spontaneous osteonecrosis of the jaws in the maxilla of mice on antiresorptive treatment: a novel ONJ mouse model. Bone 2014;68:11–9.

52. Williams DW, Lee C, Kim T, et al. Impaired bone resorption and woven bone formation are associated with development of osteonecrosis of the jaw-like lesions by bisphosphonate and anti- receptor activator of NF-κB ligand antibody in mice. Am J Pathol 2014;184:1–11.

53. Kuroshima S, Yamashita J. Chemotherapeutic and antiresorptive combination therapy suppressed lymphangiogenesis and induced osteonecrosis of the jaw-like lesions in mice. Bone 2013;56(1):101–9.

54. Allen MR, Chu TM, Ruggiero SL. Absence of exposed bone following dental extraction in beagle dogs treated with 9 months of high-dose zoledronic acid combined with dexamethasone. J Oral Maxillofac Surg 2013;71(6):1017–26.

55. Huja SS, Mason A, Fenell CE, et al. Effects of short-term zoledronic acid treatment on bone remodeling and healing at surgical sites in the maxilla and mandible of aged dogs. J Oral Maxillofac Surg 2011;69(2):418–27.

56. Allen M, Kubek D, Burr D. Cancer treatment dosing regimens of zoledronic acid result in near-complete suppression of mandible intracortical bone remodeling in beagle dogs. J Bone Miner Res 2010;25(1): 98–105.

57. Gerard DA, Carlson ER, Gotcher JE, et al. Early inhibitory effects of zoledronic acid in tooth extraction sockets in dogs are negated by recombinant human bone morphogenetic protein. J Oral Maxillofac Surg 2014;72(1):61–6.

58. Pautke C, Kreutzer K, Weitz J, et al. Bisphosphonate related osteonecrosis of the jaw: a minipig large animal model. Bone 2012;51:1–34.

59. Li Y, Xu J, Mao L, et al. Allogeneic mesenchymal stem cell therapy for bisphosphonate-related jaw osteonecrosis in Swine. Stem Cells Dev 2013;22(14): 2047–56.

60. Kikuiri T, Kim I, Yamaza T, et al. Cell-based immunotherapy with mesenchymal stem cells cures bisphosphonate-related osteonecrosis of the jaw–like disease in mice. J Bone Miner Res 2010;25(7): 1668–79.

61. Brown JP, Morin S, Leslie W, et al. Bisphosphonates for treatment of osteoporosis: expected benefits, potential harms, and drug holidays. Can Fam Physician 2014;60(4):324–33.

62. Yoshiga D, Yamashita Y, Nakamichi I, et al. Weekly teriparatide injections successfully treated advanced bisphosphonate-related osteonecrosis of the jaws. Osteoporos Int 2013;24(8):2365–9.

The Frequency of Medication-related Osteonecrosis of the Jaw and its Associated Risk Factors

CrossMark

Thomas B. Dodson, DMD, MPH

KEYWORDS

- Medication-related osteonecrosis of the jaws • Frequency • Risk factors • Zolendronate
- Oral bisphosphonates • Antiresorptive medications • Antiangiogenic agents

KEY POINTS

- Medication-related osteonecrosis of the jaws (MRONJ) is an uncommon disease among patients exposed to antiresorptive or antiangiogenic medications.
- The risk of osteonecrosis of the jaw (ONJ) among patients with cancer exposed to antiresorptive or antiangiogenic medications is about 1% (range 0.2%–6.7%).
- The risk of ONJ among patients who are managed for osteoporosis using antiresorptive medications is about 0.1% (range 0.004%–0.2%).
- Among patients exposed to oral bisphosphonates to manage osteoporosis, the risk of ONJ after tooth extraction is estimated to be 1 in 200 (0.5%).
- Among patients exposed to oral bisphosphonates to manage osteoporosis, the risk of ONJ after endodontic or periodontal surgery or implant placement is unknown.

INTRODUCTION

This article has 2 primary goals: to provide the best current frequency estimate of medication-related osteonecrosis of the jaws (MRONJ) and to identify factors associated with the risk of developing osteonecrosis of the jaw (ONJ) among patients exposed to relevant medications (ie, antiresorptive or antiangiogenic agents). Portions of this article were previously published in the 2014 update on MRONJ.[1] In the 2014 update, the review was limited to articles published through August 2012. The current article has been updated to include publications through February 2015.

Given the proliferation of data since MRONJ was originally reported in 2003, the author has applied strict inclusion criteria for the articles included in this review.[2] Inclusion criteria are:

1. Studies published between 2008 and 2015
2. Limiting studies to those with the highest levels of evidence for the available topic; that is, in descending order of validity are systematic reviews of several randomized controlled trials (RCTs) or prospective cohort studies, individual RCTs, prospective cohort studies, retrospective cohort studies, and case-control studies
3. Studies with clinical ascertainment of MRONJ

Older studies, case reports, case series, and studies that relied on medical record review or insurance-claim data to ascertain ONJ status were excluded from analyses.

How common is MRONJ? MRONJ is a serious disease whose overall frequency is low. The average general dentist may expect 1 new case of MRONJ for every 62 years in practice.[3]

Department of Oral and Maxillofacial Surgery, University of Washington School of Dentistry, 1959 Northeast Pacific Street, Health Sciences Building B-241, Box 357134, Seattle, WA 98195-7134, USA
E-mail address: tbdodson@uw.edu

Oral Maxillofacial Surg Clin N Am 27 (2015) 509–516
http://dx.doi.org/10.1016/j.coms.2015.06.003
1042-3699/15/$ – see front matter © 2015 Elsevier Inc. All rights reserved.

oralmaxsurgery.theclinics.com

To interpret MRONJ disease frequency estimates, the major consideration is the therapeutic indication for treatment, namely malignancy or osteoporosis. Disease frequency is reported herein as incidence (number of new cases per sample [or population] per unit time) or as a rate or prevalence (number of cases per sample [or population] reported as a percentage).

Challenges of Estimating the Frequency of Uncommon Diseases

Estimating disease frequency for uncommon diseases or conditions is challenging. Estimates are likely to be too large or too small relative to the true disease frequency. For example, assume that the true frequency of disease is 1:10,000 (0.01%). If one starts estimating disease frequency with the first case observed, a measurement bias is introduced. The resulting disease frequency estimate will be too high. With the first case, the disease frequency is 1:1 or 100%. After enrolling another 100 subjects, the disease frequency is now 1%. After enrolling 1000 subjects, the disease frequency estimate is 1:1000, but still a 10-fold overestimate of the true disease frequency already noted (1:10,000). In the case of MRONJ, as the sample size increases the disease frequency estimates tend to get smaller (**Table 1**).

Conversely, if the researcher starts at zero to estimate disease frequency of a rare disease, it is quite possible that after seeing 1000 subjects no cases will be encountered. The resulting disease estimate is 0% and underestimates the true disease frequency. For example, among subjects with cancer assigned to the placebo group, no cases of ONJ were identified until the sample size reached 5382.[4] The other studies that included placebo saw no cases of ONJ, and their sample sizes ranged from 903 to 1678 subjects.[5–7]

When reviewing studies that try to estimate the disease frequency of an uncommon condition such as MRONJ, readers should weight more heavily the estimates of studies composed of larger sample sizes (eg, >1000 subjects) than those estimating disease frequency with smaller sample sizes (eg, <500 subjects).

SUMMARY OF FINDINGS

Table 1 summarizes the risk of MRONJ among patients with cancer exposed to antiresorptive (oral/intravenous bisphosphonates [BPs] or denosumab) or antiangiogenic (bevacizumab) medications. The overall risk ranges from 0% to 6.7%. The bulk of the studies suggest that the risk of ONJ is in the low single digit percentages, 1% to 3%, or 1 to 3 cases per 100 patients with

cancer exposed to antiresorptive or antiangiogenic agents.

Table 2 summarizes the risk of MRONJ among patients taking antiresorptive medications (ie, oral/intravenous BPs or denosumab) for the management of osteoporosis. The overall risk for ONJ in this population ranges from 0.004% to 0.2% (4–200 cases per 100,000 subjects exposed to antiresorptive agents). The bulk of the data suggest that the risk of MRONJ is less than 0.1% (<1 per 1000 patients whose osteoporosis is being managed with antiresorptives).

RISK FACTORS FOR MEDICATION-RELATED OSTEONECROSIS OF THE JAWS

This section reviews the following risk factors for MRONJ: medications, local factors such as operations or anatomy, systemic factors such as age, sex, or other conditions, and genetic factors.

Medication-related Risk Factors

Are antiresorptive or antiangiogenic agents risk factors for osteonecrosis of the jaw?

To answer this question, we need to estimate the risk for ONJ among patients not exposed to antiresorptive or antiangiogenic medications. The risk for ONJ among patients with cancer enrolled in clinical trials and assigned to placebo groups ranges from 0% to 0.02% (0–2 cases per 10,000 patients with cancer).[4–7]

Risk for medication-related osteonecrosis of the jaws among patients with cancer

Among patients with cancer exposed to intravenous BPs, ONJ risk ranged from 0% to 6.7% (see **Table 1**).[6,8,9] The bulk of the studies suggest that the best estimate of MRONJ among patients with cancer exposed to intravenous BPs is in the low single digit percentages (1–3%).[4,10–15] One study reports the risk of ONJ among patients with cancer exposed to an oral BP (ibandronic acid) to be 0.7% in a sample of 704 subjects.[10] Among patients with cancer exposed to the antiresorptive agent, denosumab, the risk of ONJ ranged from 0.7% to 1.7%.[5,11,14,15] For patients with cancer exposed to the antiangiogenic agent, bevacizumab, one study reports the risk of ONJ to be 0.2%.[16] For patients with cancer exposed to both an intravenous BP, zoledronate, and an antiangiogenic agent, bevacizumab, Guarneri and colleagues[16] estimated the frequency of ONJ to be 0.9%. When limited to studies with level 1 evidence, namely, systematic reviews or RCTs, the risk of MRONJ in subjects exposed to zolendronate ranges from 1% to 2% (100–200 cases per 10,000 patients).[4–7,10–12,15] The risk of ONJ among

Table 1
Risk for MRONJ among patients with cancer grouped by medication

Authors,[Ref.] Year	Study Design	Medication					
		Placebo[a]	IV BP[b]	Oral BP[c]	Denosumab	Bevacizumab	Bevacizumab and Zolendronate
Gnant et al,[6] 2015	RCT	0% (903)	0% (900)	—	—	—	—
Barrett-Lee et al,[10] 2014	RCT	—	1.3% (697)	0.7% (704)	—	—	—
Coleman et al,[7] 2014	RCT	0% (1678)	1.7% (1681)	—	—	—	—
Qi et al,[5] 2014	Systematic review	0% (1450)	1.1% (2928)	—	1.7% (4585)	—	—
Henry et al,[11] 2014	RCT	—	1.1% (792)	—	0.8% (786)	—	—
Jackson et al,[12] 2014	RCT	—	3.7% (981)	—	—	—	—
Chiang et al,[8] 2013	Prospective cohort study	—	0% (414)	—	—	—	—
Van den Wyngaert et al,[13] 2013	Prospective cohort study	—	6% (298)	—	—	—	—
Scagliotti et al,[15] 2012	RCT	—	0.8% (400)	—	0.7% (411)	—	—
Guarneri et al,[16] 2010	Systematic review	—	—	—	—	0.2% (1076)	0.9% (233)
Stopeck et al,[14] 2010	RCT	—	2.0% (1020)	—	1.4% (1013)	—	—
Vahtsevanos et al,[9] 2009	Prospective cohort study	—	6.7% (1163)	—	—	—	—
Mauri et al,[4] 2009	Systematic review	0.02% (5382)	0.3% (3987)	—	—	—	—

Abbreviations: BP, bisphosphonate; IV, intravenous; RCT, randomized controlled clinical trial.
[a] Sample size in parentheses.
[b] Zolendronate.
[c] Oral ibandronic acid.
Data from Refs.[4–12,14–16]

Table 2
Risk of MRONJ among subjects treated for osteoporosis grouped by medication

Authors,[Ref.] Year	Study Design	Placebo	Zolendronate	Oral BP	Denosumab
Sugimoto et al,[20] 2014	RCT	—	—	—	0.1% (775)[a]
Bone et al,[19] 2013	RCT	—	—	—	—
Long-term exposure group (6 y)	—	—	—	—	0.2% (2342)
Short-term exposure group (2 y)	—	—	—	—	0.1% (2207)
Papapoulos et al,[17] 2012	RCT	0% (3383)	—	—	0.04% (4549)
Grbic et al,[18] 2010	Systematic review	0.02% (4945)	0.02% (5864)	—	—
Malden and Lopes,[24] 2012	Prospective cohort study	—	—	0.004% (900,000)	—
Lo et al,[22] 2010	Cross-sectional	—	—	0.1%[b] (8572)	—

[a] Sample size in parentheses.
[b] Prevalence estimate. All other estimates reported in the table are incidence rates.
Data from Refs.[17–20,22,24]

patients with cancer exposed to zolendronate is about 50 to 100 times higher than in patients with cancer treated with placebo.

Among patients with cancer exposed to denosumab, a RANK-L inhibitor, the risk of MRONJ in studies with level 1 evidence ranges from 0.7% to 1.7%.[5,11,14,15] The risk of ONJ for patients with cancer exposed to denosumab approximates the risk in patients with cancer exposed to zolendronate and is about 50 times higher than the risk for ONJ in patients with cancer exposed to placebo.

The risk for MRONJ among patients with cancer exposed to bevacizumab, an antiangiogenic agent, is 0.2% (20 cases per 10,000).[16] The risk may be higher among patients exposed to both bevacizumab and zolendronate, 0.9% (90 cases per 10,000).[16]

Risk for medication-related osteonecrosis of the jaws among patients treated for osteoporosis

Among patients with osteoporosis exposed to placebo agents, the risk for ONJ ranges from 0% to 0.02% (0–2 cases per 10,000 subjects) **(Table 2)**.[17,18]

For those patients with osteoporosis exposed to zolendronate, the risk for MRONJ is 0.02% (2 cases per 10,000 subjects) and approximates the risk for ONJ in osteoporotic patients exposed to placebo.[18]

For subjects with osteoporosis exposed to denosumab, the risk for MRONJ ranges from 0.04% to 0.2% (4–20 cases per 10,000 subjects).[17,19,20]

Most clinicians see patients exposed to oral BPs for the management of osteoporosis. In 2008, 5.1 million patients older than 55 years received a prescription for a BP. A recent Federal study estimated that the prevalence of BP exposure was 7 for every 100 persons in the United States who received a prescription for a BP in the outpatient setting.[21] Ironically, the studies estimating MRONJ risk in this patient population have the weakest levels of evidence of the various study groups, for example, survey or retrospective cohort studies with ascertainment of disease based on a combination of examination or review of medical records.

In a cross-sectional survey study of more than 13,000 Kaiser-Permanente members, the prevalence of ONJ in patients receiving long-term oral BP therapy was reported at 0.1% (10 cases per 10,000).[22] Felsenberg and Hoffmeister[23] reported a prevalence of MRONJ among patients treated with BPs for osteoporosis of 0.0004% (<1 case per 100,000 exposed), based on reports of 3 cases to the German Central Registry of Necrosis of the Jaw. In a more recent report, Malden and Lopes[24] derived an incidence of 0.004% (0.4 cases per 10,000 patient-years of exposure to alendronate) from 11 cases of MRONJ reported in a population of 900,000 people living in southeast Scotland.

Based on a case-control study, the risk of ONJ was 13.1 times greater among patients exposed to oral BPs than in a unexposed counterparts (P<.001).[25] No cases of ONJ were identified among subjects exposed to intravenous BPs.

Regardless of indications for therapy, the duration of antiresorptive therapy is a risk factor for developing ONJ. Among patients with cancer exposed to zolendronate or denosumab, the incidence of developing ONJ was 0.6% and 0.5% at 1 year, 0.9% and 1.1% at 2 years, and 1.3% and 1.1% at 3 years, respectively.[11] In this study, the risk for ONJ among subjects exposed to denosumab plateaued between years 2 and 3. In a study by Saad and colleagues[26] the investigators combined 3 blinded phase 3 trials and found similar results, including a plateau after 2 years for patients exposed to denosumab.

For patients receiving oral BP therapy to manage osteoporosis, the prevalence of ONJ increases over time from near 0 at baseline to 0.2% after 4 or more years of BP exposure.[27] The median duration of BP exposure for patients exposed to oral BP was 4.4 years. For patients without ONJ, the median exposure to oral BPs was 3.5 years.

Although the data are more limited, a similar phenomenon was noted in osteoporotic subjects exposed to denosumab. After 2 years of exposure, the incidence of ONJ was 0.09% and doubled to 0.2% after 6 years of exposure to denosumab.[19]

In summary, when compared with patients with cancer receiving antiresorptive treatment, the risk of ONJ for patients whose osteoporosis is being managed using oral BPs or denosumab is about 10 times smaller (0.1%). The risk of ONJ is about 100 times smaller for those patients receiving intravenous zoledronate for managing osteoporosis in comparison with patients with cancer receiving intravenous zoledronate.

Local Factors

Operative treatment

Among patients with MRONJ, dentoalveolar surgery is the most common risk factor, with tooth extraction being the most common predisposing event ranging from 52% to 61%.[9,26,28] In a case-control study among patients with cancer exposed to zoledronate, tooth extraction was associated with a 16-fold increased risk for ONJ when compared with counterparts without ONJ (odds ratio [OR] = 16.4; 95% confidence interval [CI] 3.4–79.6).[29] In a longitudinal cohort study, in a sample of patients with cancer exposed to intravenous BPs (predominately zolendronate), tooth extraction was associated with a 33-fold increased risk for ONJ.[9]

It is critical to exercise caution in interpreting tooth extraction as the causal precipitant of MRONJ that develops after the extraction. Tooth extraction may be incidental to the disease rather than a precipitant of the disease. Dental pain and other inflammatory symptoms mimic symptoms

manifested by necrotic bone. As such, pain and localized swelling or drainage diagnosed as having an odontogenic source may be a misdiagnosis when, in fact, the source is necrotic bone.

Among patients with MRONJ, it is helpful to know how often tooth extraction was a preceding event. However, this is not what patients or clinicians want to know; rather, they wish to know: "Among patients exposed to antiresorptive or antiangiogenic medications, what is the risk for developing ONJ following tooth extraction?" The best current estimate for the risk of ONJ among patients exposed to oral BPs following tooth extraction is 0.5%.[30] This estimate was derived from a prospective evaluation of 194 patients exposed to oral BPs who underwent extraction of 1 or more teeth. In this sample, 1 patient developed ONJ after tooth extraction. In a retrospective cohort study composed of a sample of 99 subjects undergoing tooth extraction after exposure to oral BPs, 1 patient (1%) developed ONJ.[31]

Estimates for developing ONJ after tooth extraction among patients with cancer exposed to intravenous BPs range from 1.6% to 14.8%. In a retrospective cohort study, in a sample of patients with cancer exposed to zolendronate (n = 27), 4 (14.8%) subjects developed ONJ after extraction.[31] In prospective cohort study composed of 176 subjects with cancer and exposed to zolendronate, 5 subjects (2.8%) developed ONJ.[32] In a prospective cohort study of 63 subjects who underwent extraction of at least 1 tooth with a history of cancer and exposure to intravenous BPs, 1 subject (1.6%) developed ONJ.[33] Among these aforementioned studies, the findings from the prospective studies should be weighted more heavily because of their larger sample sizes and study design.

The risk of developing ONJ among patients who have been exposed to antiresorptive or antiangiogenic medications for other dentoalveolar operations such as dental implant, root-end endodontic, or periodontal procedures is unknown. When advising patients regarding risk for these procedures, the author uses the risk of ONJ following tooth extraction (0.5%).

Anatomic factors

Limited new information regarding anatomic risk factors for MRONJ is available. MRONJ is more likely to appear in the mandible (73%) than the maxilla (22.5%), and can appear in both jaws (4.5%).[26] Denture use was associated with an increased risk for ONJ among patients with cancer exposed to zolendronate (OR = 4.9; 95% CI 1.2–20.1).[29] In another study by Vahtsevanos and colleagues,[9] in a sample of 1621 patients with cancer treated with intravenous zoledronate, ibandronate, or pamidronate there was a 2-fold increased risk for ONJ among denture wearers.

Concomitant oral disease

Preexisting inflammatory dental disease such as periodontal disease or periapical disorder is a recognized risk factor.[31,34] Among patients with cancer with MRONJ, preexisting inflammatory dental disease was a risk factor in 50% of the cases.[26,31] Given that a common treatment of inflammatory dental disease is tooth extraction, it is unclear whether the preexisting dental disease confounds the relationship between tooth extraction and risk for MRONJ. It would be valuable to see an estimate of the association between tooth extraction and MRONJ adjusted for preexisting inflammatory dental disease. Likewise, discriminating between pain from an odontogenic versus necrotic bone source can be difficult.

Demographic and Systemic Factors and Other Medication Factors

Age and sex are variably reported as risk factors for MRONJ.[9,26,29,31,34–36] Comorbid conditions among patients with cancer inconsistently reported to be a risk factor associated with an increased risk for MRONJ include anemia (hemoglobin <10 g/dL) and diabetes.[25,27,34,37] Cancer type is also variably reported as a risk factor.[5,9]

Corticosteroids are associated with an increased risk for MRONJ.[26,34] Antiangiogenic agents, when given in addition to antiresorptive medications, are associated with an increased risk of ONJ.[16,26]

Tobacco use is variably reported as a risk factor for MRONJ. In a case-control study, tobacco use was near statistically significantly ($P = .09$) associated with ONJ in patients with cancer (OR = 3.0; 95% CI 0.8–10.4).[29] Borromeo and colleagues[25] reported an association between tobacco use and ONJ, with an OR of 5.5 (95% CI 1.3–22.9) that was statistically significant ($P = .02$). Tsao and colleagues[34] reported in a case-control study that tobacco use was not associated with ONJ in a sample of patients with cancer exposed to zolendronate. Vahtsevanos and colleagues[9] also did not report an association between tobacco use and MRONJ.

Genetic Factors

As noted earlier, if a clinician extracts teeth in 200 patients exposed to oral BPs, 199 patients do well and 1 develops MRONJ.[30] In the setting of rare diseases or conditions, phenotypic, operative, or systemic risk factors are insufficiently sensitive to predict which 1 of the 200 patients having tooth extractions will develop MRONJ. As such, there may be value in identifying genetic risk factors associated with developing MRONJ. Recent studies have identified single nucleotide polymorphisms (SNPs) associated with MRONJ.[38–43] Most of the SNP variability has been noted in genes associated with bone turnover or collagen formation. In addition to predicting patients most likely to develop MRONJ, the genetic approach may offer insights into the basic physiologic or metabolic pathways associated with MRONJ.

SUMMARY

MRONJ is a serious complication of treating patients with cancer or managing patients with osteoporosis. It is an uncommon complication whose manifestations range from asymptomatic to requiring extensive operative treatment and adversely affecting patients' qualify of life. This review reconfirms that antiresorptive medications such as oral or intravenous BPs and denosumab are the most common risk factors for developing ONJ. The risk of MRONJ is greater in patients with cancer than in those receiving antiresorptive treatments for osteoporosis by a factor of 10. Whether this is due to the relative immunosuppressed state of patients with cancer or their greater exposure to potent antiresorptive medications in terms of dose and frequency is unclear. A major opportunity for advancement in the prediction and understanding of MRONJ is through pharmacoepidemiology.[44]

REFERENCES

1. Ruggiero SL, Dodson TB, Fantasia J, et al. American Association of Oral and Maxillofacial Surgeons position paper on medication-related osteonecrosis of the jaw. 2014 Update. J Oral Maxillofac Surg 2014; 72:1938–56.

2. Marx RE. Pamidronate (Aredia) and zoledronate (Zometa) induced avascular necrosis of the jaws: a growing epidemic. J Oral Maxillofac Surg 2003;61: 1115.

3. Ulmner M, Jarnbring F, Torring O. Osteonecrosis of the jaw in Sweden associated with the oral use of bisphosphonate. J Oral Maxillofac Surg 2014;72:76–82.

4. Mauri D, Valachis A, Polyzos IP, et al. Osteonecrosis of the jaw and use of bisphosphonates in adjuvant breast cancer treatment: a meta-analysis. Breast Cancer Res Treat 2009;116:433.

5. Qi W-K, Tang L-N, He A-N, et al. Risk of osteonecrosis of the jaw in cancer patients receiving denosumab: a meta-analysis of seven randomized controlled trials. Int J Clin Oncol 2014;19:403–10.

6. Gnant M, Mlineritsch B, Stoeger H, et al. Zolendronic acid combined with adjuvant endocrine therapy of tamoxifen versus anastrozol plus ovarian function suppression in premenopausal early breast cancer: final analysis of the Austrian Breast and Colorectal Cancer Study Group Trial 12. Ann Oncol 2015;26: 313–20.

7. Coleman R, Cameron D, Dodwell D, et al. Adjuvant zoledronic acid in patients with early breast cancer: Final efficacy analysis of the AZURE (BIG 01/04) randomized open-label phase 3 trial. Lancet Oncol 2014;15:997–1006.

8. Chiang P-H, Wang H-C, Lai Y-L, et al. Zoledronic acid treatment for cancerous bone metastases: a phase IV study in Taiwan. J Cancer Res Ther 2013; 9:653–9.

9. Vahtsevanos K, Kyrgidis A, Verrou E, et al. Longitudinal cohort study of risk factors in cancer patients of bisphosphonate-related osteonecrosis of the jaw. J Clin Oncol 2009;27:5356.

10. Barrett-Lee P, Casbard A, Abraham J, et al. Oral ibandronic acid versus intravenous zoledronic acid in treatment of bone metastases from breast cancer: a randomized, open label, non-inferiority phase 3 trial. Lancet Oncol 2014;15:114–22.

11. Henry D, Vadhan-Raj S, Hirsh V, et al. Delaying skeletal-related events in a randomized phase 3 study of denosumab versus zoledronic acid in patients with advanced cancer: an analysis of data from patients with solid tumors. Support Care Cancer 2013;22:679–87.

12. Jackson GH, Morgan GJ, Davies FE, et al. Osteonecrosis of the jaw and renal safety in patients with newly diagnosed multiple myeloma: Medical Research Council Myeloma IX Study results. Br J Haematol 2014;166:109–17.

13. Van den Wyngaert T, Delforge M, Doye C, et al. Prospective observational study of treatment pattern, effectiveness and safety of zoledronic acid therapy beyond 24 months in patients with multiple myeloma or bone metastases from solid tumors. Support Care Cancer 2013;21:3483–90.

14. Stopeck AT, Lipton A, Body JJ, et al. Denosumab compared with zoledronic acid for the treatment of bone metastases in patients with advanced breast cancer: a randomized, double-blind study. J Clin Oncol 2010;28:5132–9.

15. Scagliotti GV, Hirsh V, Siena S, et al. Overall survival improvement in patients with lung cancer and bone metastases treated with denosumab versus zoledronic acid: subgroup analysis from a randomized phase 3 study. J Thorac Oncol 2012;7:1823.

16. Guarneri V, Miles D, Robert N, et al. Bevacizumab and osteonecrosis of the jaw: incidence and association with bisphosphonate therapy in three large prospective trials in advanced breast cancer. Breast Cancer Res Treat 2010;122:181.

17. Papapoulos S, Chapurlat R, Libanati C, et al. Five years of denosumab exposure in women with postmenopausal osteoporosis: results from the first two years of the FREEDOM extension. J Bone Miner Res 2012;27:694.

18. Grbic JT, Black DM, Lyles KW, et al. The incidence of osteonecrosis of the jaw in patients receiving 5 milligrams of zoledronic acid: data from the health outcomes and reduced incidence with zoledronic acid once yearly clinical trials program. J Am Dent Assoc 2010;141:1365.

19. Bone HG, Chapurlat R, Brandi M-L, et al. The effect of three or six years of denosumab exposure in women with postmenopausal osteoporosis: Results from the FREEDOM extension. J Clin Endocrinol Metab 2013;98:4483–92.

20. Sugimoto T, Matsumoto T, Hosoi T, et al. Three-year denosumab treatment in postmenopausal women and men with osteoporosis: results from a 1-year open-label extension of the Denosumab Fracture Intervention Randomized Placebo Controlled Trial (DIRECT). Osteoporos Int 2014;26(2):765–74.

21. Background document for meeting of Advisory Committee for Reproductive Health Drugs and Drug Safety and Risk Management Advisory Committee. Prepared by Division of Reproductive and Urologic Products, Office of New Drugs, Division of Pharmacovigilance II, Office of Surveillance and Epidemiology, Division of Epidemiology, Office of Surveillance and Epidemiology, Center for Drug Evaluation and Research, Food and Drug Administration, September 9, 2011. p. 14. Available at: http://www.fda.gov/AdvisoryCommittees/CommitteesMeetingMaterials/Drugs/DrugSafetyand RiskManagementAdvisoryCommittee/ucm270957. htm. Accessed February 6, 2015.

22. Lo JC, O'Ryan FS, Gordon NP, et al. Prevalence of osteonecrosis of the jaw in patients with oral bisphosphonate exposure. J Oral Maxillofac Surg 2010;68:243.

23. Felsenberg D, Hoffmeister B. Necrosis of the jaw after high-dose bisphosphonate therapy. Kiefernekrosen nach hoch dosierter Bisphosphonattherapie. Dtsch Arztebl 2006;103:3078.

24. Malden N, Lopes V. An epidemiological study of alendronate-related osteonecrosis of the jaws. A case series from the south-east of Scotland with attention given to case definition and prevalence. J Bone Miner Metab 2012;30:171.

25. Borromeo GL, Brand C, Clement JG, et al. A large case-control study reveals a positive association between bisphosphonate use and delayed dental healing and osteonecrosis of the jaw. J Bone Miner Res 2014;29:1363–8.

26. Saad F, Brown JE, Van Poznak C, et al. Incidence, risk factors, and outcomes of osteonecrosis of the jaw: integrated analysis from three blinded

active-controlled phase III trials in cancer patients with bone metastases. Ann Oncol 2012;23:1341.

27. Frequency of ONJ over time. Available at: http://www.fda.gov/AdvisoryCommittees/CommitteesMeetingMaterials/Drugs/DrugSafetyandRiskManagementAdvisoryCommittee/ucm270957.htm. Accessed February 6, 2015. p. 19.

28. Fehm T, Beck V, Banys M, et al. Bisphosphonate-induced osteonecrosis of the jaw (ONJ): Incidence and risk factors in patients with breast cancer and gynecological malignancies. Gynecol Oncol 2009;112:605.

29. Kyrgidis A, Vahtsevanos K, Koloutsos G, et al. Bisphosphonate-related osteonecrosis of the jaws: a case-control study of risk factors in breast cancer patients. J Clin Oncol 2008;26:4634.

30. Kunchur R, Need A, Hughes T, et al. Clinical investigation of C-terminal cross-linking telopeptide test in prevention and management of bisphosphonate-associated osteonecrosis of the jaws. J Oral Maxillofac Surg 2009;67:1167.

31. Yamazaki T, Yamori M, Ishizaki T, et al. Increased incidence of osteonecrosis of the jaw after tooth extraction in patients treated with bisphosphonates: a cohort study. Int J Oral Maxillofac Surg 2012;41:1397.

32. Mozzati M, Arata V, Gallesio G. Tooth extraction in patients on zoledronic acid therapy. Oral Oncol 2012;48:817.

33. Scoletta M, Arata V, Arduino PG, et al. Tooth extractions in intravenous bisphosphonate-treated patients: a refined protocol. J Oral Maxillofac Surg 2013;71:994.

34. Tsao C, Darby I, Ebeling PR, et al. Oral health risk factors for bisphosphonate-associated jaw osteonecrosis. J Oral Maxillofac Surg 2013;71:1360.

35. Kharazmi M, Hallberg P, Michaelsson K. Gender related difference in the risk of bisphosphonate associated atypical femoral fracture and osteonecrosis of the jaw. Ann Rheum Dis 2014;73:1594.

36. Hennedige AA, Jayasinghe J, Khajeh J, et al. Systematic review of the incidence of bisphosphonate related osteonecrosis of the jaw in children diagnosed with osteogenesis imperfecta. J Oral Maxillofac Res 2013;4:e1.

37. Peer A, Khamaisi M. Diabetes as a risk factor for medication-related osteonecrosis of the jaw. J Dent Res 2015;94:252–60.

38. Katz J, Gong Y, Salmasinia D, et al. Genetic polymorphisms and other risk factors associated with bisphosphonate induced osteonecrosis of the jaw. Int J Oral Maxillofac Surg 2011;40:605.

39. Nicoletti P, Cartsos VM, Palaska PK, et al. Genome-wide pharmacogenetics of bisphosphonate-induced osteonecrosis of the jaw: the role of RBMS3. Oncologist 2012;17:279.

40. Marini F, Tonelli P, Cavalli L, et al. Pharmacogenetics of bisphosphonate-associated osteonecrosis of the jaw. Front Biosci (Elite Ed) 2011;3:364.

41. Balla B, Vaszilko M, Kosa JP, et al. New approach to analyze genetic and clinical data in bisphosphonate-induces osteonecrosis of the jaw. Oral Dis 2012;18:580–5.

42. La Ferla F, Paolicchi E, Crea F, et al. An aromatase polymorphism (g.132810C>T) predicts risk of bisphosphonate-related osteonecrosis of the jaw. Biomark Med 2012;6:210–9.

43. Zhong D-N, Wu J-Z, Li G-J. Association between CYP2C8 (rs1934951) polymorphism and bisphosphonate-related osteonecrosis of the jaws in patients on bisphosphonate therapy: a meta-analysis. Acta Haematol 2013;129:90–5.

44. Kim J-H, Ko YJ, Kim J-Y, et al. Genetic investigation of bisphosphonate-related osteonecrosis of the jaw (BRONJ) via whole exome sequencing and bioinformatics. PLos One 2015;10:e0118084.

Management of Medication-Related Osteonecrosis of the Jaw

William Bradford Williams, DMD, MD, Felice O'Ryan, DDS*

KEYWORDS

- MRONJ • Bisphosphonate • Denosumab • Oral surgery • Maxillofacial surgery • BRONJ

KEY POINTS

- Treatment of medication-related osteonecrosis of the jaw (MRONJ) should be based on the patient's symptoms, comorbidities, and goals.
- Collaboration with members of the patient's dental and medical team is encouraged.
- Effective medical management of MRONJ includes topical and oral antimicrobials, pentoxifylline, and vitamin E.
- Plain films are inadequate for surgical planning.
- Successful surgery is predicated on primary wound closure and complete excision of necrotic bone.

INTRODUCTION

Medication-related osteonecrosis of the jaw (MRONJ) was first reported in 2003 and primarily involved patients receiving intravenous bisphosphonates for treatment of skeletal-related malignancies.[1] Soon thereafter, similar cases involving oral bisphosphonates and denosumab began appearing. Although the mechanism of action of these drugs may differ, both involve osteoclast inhibition and disruption of normal bone turnover and healing.[2]

There is no consensus regarding the clinical management of patients with MRONJ. Among the reasons for this are an incomplete understanding of the etiopathogenesis of the disease and the difficulty in defining successful treatment. Successful treatment may be that which results in a cure, with complete mucosal coverage and elimination of disease, or that which improves the quality of life

without a cure (palliation). The American Association of Oral and Maxillofacial Surgery 2014 *Position Paper on Medication-Related Osteonecrosis of the Jaws* states that the "Treatment objectives for patients with an established diagnosis of MRONJ are to eliminate pain, control infection of the soft and hard tissue, and minimize the progression or occurrence of bone necrosis."[3] Additionally, we feel that helping patients to understand the chronicity and potential progression of the disease is essential to a satisfactory outcome.

The aim of this review is to share our treatment approach to patients with MRONJ once the diagnosis has been made. Fundamentally, treatment can be divided into medical and surgical therapies, although a combination is often used. For purposes of clarity, when referring to disease stage in this review we employ the staging system as described in the 2014 American Association of Oral and Maxillofacial Surgery position paper.[3]

Division Maxillofacial Surgery, Oakland Medical Center, Kaiser Permanente, 3600 Broadway Kaiser, Oakland, CA 94611, USA
* Corresponding author.
E-mail address: Felice.O'Ryan@kp.org

Oral Maxillofacial Surg Clin N Am 27 (2015) 517–525
http://dx.doi.org/10.1016/j.coms.2015.06.007
1042-3699/15/$ – see front matter © 2015 Elsevier Inc. All rights reserved.

MEDICAL MANAGEMENT

In our practice, treatment of MRONJ with medical therapy alone is most commonly employed for patients with less severe disease, those who decline surgery, or those whose comorbidities preclude them from surgery. Medical therapies currently in use include topical, oral and intravenous antimicrobials, other medications and hyperbaric oxygen (HBO).

Antimicrobials

Topical antimicrobials

Chlorhexidine gluconate 0.12% is a topical bactericidal and bacteriostatic agent[4–6] that has been shown to be effective in treatment of patients with MRONJ.[3,7] Although the pathogenesis of MRONJ remains unclear, there is evidence that the oral flora, and more specifically biofilms, contribute to the disease process.[8] The use of chlorhexidine is thus rationalized by its ability to decrease total bacterial counts, including potentially pathologic organisms. Advantages of chlorhexidine include low cost, ease of use, availability, patient acceptance, and efficacy. Disadvantages include patient intolerance, lack of compliance associated with long-term use, dental staining, and opportunistic infection, as well as alterations in taste. In our practice, we commonly recommend chlorhexidine for management of stage 1 disease as a singular therapy (**Fig. 1**). For more advanced stages, we routinely recommend chlorhexidine in addition to other medical and surgical therapies.

Oral antimicrobials

Antimicrobials are a mainstay in the management of MRONJ.[3,7,9,10] Antimicrobial therapy is based on clinical observation and scientific literature suggesting that pathogenic bacteria may contribute to MRONJ. The precise organism(s) responsible remain to be identified but it seems that most infections are polymicrobial.[3,11,12] Systemic antibiotics may decrease bacterial counts in the oral cavity, including pathogenic organisms. Selection of specific antibiotics should be based on patient tolerance, compliance, and prior antibiotic exposure. One should also consider therapies targeted against common colonizers of MRONJ lesions, including Actinobacteria, Firmicutes, Fusobacteria, and Bacteroidetes.[13–15] Members of these phyla include aerobic and anaerobic organisms commonly susceptible to penicillin; therefore, penicillin remains our first antibiotic choice. Our most common penicillin alternates are clindamycin, fluoroquinolones, and/or metronidazole (**Fig. 2**). Although there are no data to clarify the most appropriate duration of antibiotic therapy for MRONJ, we generally prescribe a 2-week course for patients with persistent stage 1 disease and up to a 4- to 6-week course for more severe cases.

Intravenous antimicrobials

Intravenous antimicrobials may be of benefit in patients with pathogenic organisms resistant to oral agents and may provide greater tissue penetration in certain cases. However, there have been no satisfactory trials demonstrating greater efficacy of intravenous agents compared with oral medications in management of MRONJ.[16,17] When all available oral agents have been exhausted and no less invasive option exists, it is our practice to employ long-term (6 weeks) intravenous antimicrobials. In the future, it is conceivable that antimicrobial therapy may be more effective in MRONJ treatment when combined with developing delivery mechanisms most capable of penetrating biofilms.

Other Medications

Pentoxifylline and vitamin E

The combination of pentoxifylline and vitamin E has been used successfully in the treatment of jaw osteoradionecrosis and MRONJ; however, the specific mechanism of action in MRONJ remains unclear.[18–22] Pentoxifylline (Trental), a xanthine derivative with an excellent safety profile, is used primarily for the treatment of intermittent

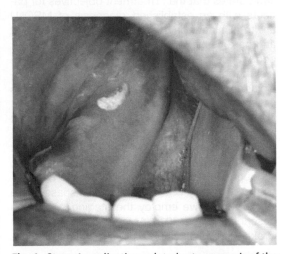

Fig. 1. Stage 1 medication-related osteonecrosis of the jaw of the right alveolar ridge, which was asymptomatic but noted on routine dental examination after dental extractions. There was no exposed bone in the extraction sites. The patient had a 12-year history of oral bisphosphonate exposure for treatment of osteoporosis and no other comorbidities. Treatment included chlorhexidine oral rinses and routine oral hygiene practices. Resolution of the lesion was seen at 3 months.

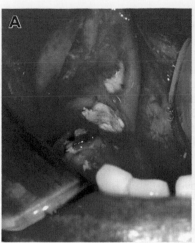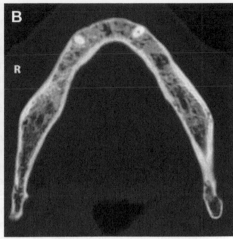

Fig. 2. (*A*) Stage 2 medication-related osteonecrosis of the jaw (MRONJ) in the right mandible of a 77-year-old man with multiple myeloma and a 12-month history of pamidronate exposure. His comorbidities included diabetes mellitus, end-stage renal disease, and gout. He presented with several areas of painful exposed bone in the right mandibular alveolus that developed after wearing a poorly fitting partial denture. (*B*) CT demonstrates bony sclerosis in the area but no bony sequestra. Treatment consisted of oral antibiotic therapy (clindamycin because the patient was allergic to penicillin) and chlorhexidine rinses. The patient died with stage 2 MRONJ several months after diagnosis.

claudication and other symptoms of peripheral vascular disease. It has been shown to decrease inflammation and reduce blood viscosity by increasing erythrocyte deformability.[23] Vitamin E decreases tissue inflammation and fibrosis, and is a scavenger of free radicals capable of cellular injury.[19] Alpha tocopherol is the most active form of vitamin E in humans, and is widely available, well-tolerated, and readily absorbed. Numerous reports supporting the role of both inflammation and decreased vascularity as contributors to MRONJ make the use of this relatively well-tolerated drug combination a rational choice.[3] The duration of treatment has not been clarified, but borrowing from the osteoradionecrosis literature benefits may plateau after 2 to 3 years of use.[22,24] Our group typically offers this therapy to any patient regardless of disease stage. The recommended dose of pentoxifylline is 400 mg sustained release twice daily and 1000 IU vitamin E daily. Reasons for termination of therapy include patient intolerance, disease resolution, or after 36 months. However, because treatment duration remains empiric continued administration should be determined by the patient, treating physician, and medical team. In addition, we routinely maintain these medications perioperatively in those who require surgical treatment of the MRONJ.

Teriparatide

Teriparatide (Forteo) is a subcutaneously administered drug used primarily in the treatment of osteoporosis. The drug is composed of 34 amino acids of the *N*-terminal chain of parathyroid hormone and retains the anabolic effects of endogenous parathyroid hormone, including promotion of bone remodeling. Its use in MRONJ treatment began when osteoporotic patients with bisphosphonate-associated MRONJ had their osteoporosis therapy changed to teriparatide and resolution of their oral lesions was noted.[25] There is also a case report of intravenous bisphosphonate-related MRONJ resolving after teriparatide administration.[26] Teriparatide is thought to stimulate effectively osteoblast function and proliferation, increase osseous cell signaling (including Wnt), and activate osteoclasts.[27]

At the time of this publication, there are several case reports but few well-controlled studies to demonstrate the efficacy of this medication.[10,25,26,28] The safety, side effects, dosing, and duration of therapy for the management of MRONJ are not known. Currently, we have not used this agent in our practice for treatment of MRONJ and it is important to note that teriparatide is contraindicated in patients with metastatic bone disease or osteosarcoma. Certainly, promising results have been observed with this therapy and, given the limited options available for treatment of MRONJ, its use should be considered and studied further.

Hyperbaric Oxygen Therapy

HBO therapy has been used for management of osteoradionecrosis of the jaw for many years and more recently has been applied to treatment of MRONJ.[3,10,29] Those advocating HBO for treatment of MRONJ argue that HBO provides greater oxygen to tissues with impaired vascularization. Additionally, HBO reverses impaired leukocyte function and also supplies reactive oxygen and nitrogen species. All of these effects theoretically contribute to improved wound healing and bone turnover. HBO is seldom used as a singular treatment modality, but is more commonly used as a surgical adjunct. Freiberger and colleagues[29,30] demonstrated slightly greater healing in patients who received HBO after surgical debridement (52%) compared with those who underwent only surgical debridement (33%), but this difference was not statistically significant ($P = .203$). In summary, the clinical utility of HBO for management of MRONJ remains unclear and for this reason we rarely use it for our patients. HBO therapy is a controversial, costly, and time-intensive treatment whose efficacy deserves further study.

SURGICAL MANAGEMENT

Our focus in the surgical treatment of MRONJ is directed toward stage-specific therapeutic options. Patients with stage 0 and stage 1 disease generally do not warrant surgical intervention, but benefit from medical management, as outlined elsewhere in this article. In our practice, surgical treatment is offered when disease progresses to the point where symptoms are not controlled with medical therapies. Regardless of disease stage any overtly mobile necrotic bony sequestra should always be removed.

A wide spectrum of disease is often seen with stage 2 MRONJ, ranging from focal minimally symptomatic exposed bone to severely painful widespread bone necrosis. It is thus difficult to recommend a single surgical treatment approach in these patients. Rather, the decision regarding operative intervention depends on the patient's medical status, comorbidities, pain level, their treatment goals, and the extent of disease. Those with mild stage 2 disease who have minimal pain and localized bone exposure may not require surgical intervention and may remain stable with medical management. A number of surgical treatment modalities, all with varying success rates, have been described for patients with symptomatic stage 2 MRONJ.

Debridement and marginal and segmental resection are terms commonly seen in the literature describing surgical treatment of MRONJ. Debridement and marginal resection both refer to removal of necrotic bone, primarily in the alveolus, with the goal of maintaining an intact inferior border of the mandible. Segmental resection, on the other hand, refers to en bloc removal of involved bone, including the inferior border of the mandible, with a resulting continuity defect. Success rates vary widely in response to local debridement/marginal resection ranging from 15% to 100%.[10] Higher success rates have been found when debridement was combined with multilayer primary soft tissue closure and failure to achieve adequate soft tissue closure has been thought to affect surgical outcomes adversely.[31–33] Success of debridement or marginal resection may also be limited by the difficulty in differentiating healthy from diseased bone. Inadequate removal of affected bone has been found to increase MRONJ recurrence.[34,35]

Because the extent of the osteonecrosis is often greater than what is seen clinically, preoperative imaging with CT or cone beam CT, bone scintigraphy, and/or MRI can also aid in determining the type and extent of surgery and assist in identifying bony margins.[36–38]

Intraoperative fluorescence-guided debridement has been suggested to assist in differentiating necrotic from viable bone.[39–43] Tetracycline is used as a bone label for this purpose because it is incorporated into sites of bone remodeling and thus will only be seen in viable bone. The technique involves preoperative administration of doxycycline (100 mg twice a day 10 days before surgery). A fluorescent light source is applied to the affected region during debridement and areas of necrotic bone are seen to fluoresce as a pale bluish-white color whereas viable bone appears brightly fluorescent.[41] Autofluorescence (using the fluorescent lamp without preoperative administration of doxycycline) has also been reported to aid with the identification of viable bone.[43]

During surgical debridement, extraction of any involved teeth is also indicated. It is better to debride diseased tissue adequately, including removing adjacent potentially involved teeth, than it is to leave the area inadequately treated to preserve teeth. Any sharp bony spicules should be removed and extraction sockets and bony margins should be free of sharp edges to aid in achieving tension-free primary closure.

All resected hard and soft tissue should be sent for histopathologic examination as well as culture and sensitivities to allow directed postoperative antibiotic therapy. Bedogni and colleagues[34] noted that recurrent MRONJ was seen in those cases where bony margins showed chronic osteomyelitis indicating inadequate removal of diseased tissue.

Adjunctive treatments, including autologous platelet-rich plasma and low-level laser therapy, have been used in conjunction with surgical debridement to improve postoperative healing.[10,44,45] The data are inconclusive as to the added value of these modalities. A systematic review of the literature on autologous platelet concentrates concluded that, although the evidence was weak, the addition of platelet concentrates improved healing outcomes after surgical debridement of osteonecrosis.[44]

Low-level laser therapy, purported to stimulate bone healing by increasing vascularity and osteoblastic differentiation, has been used in conjunction with surgical debridement of osteonecrosis.[46,47] However, rates of healing after surgical debridement with and without low-level laser therapy are comparable and further research is needed to determine the value of low-level laser therapy.[10,48–50]

In summary, in cases of stage 2 MRONJ when debridement and marginal resection is determined

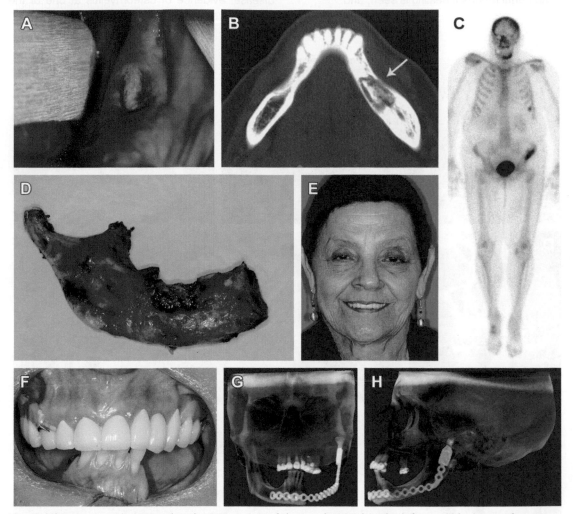

Fig. 3. (A) Stage 3 medication-related osteonecrosis of the jaw (MRONJ) in the left mandible 1 year after extraction of left mandibular second molar tooth in a 57-year-old woman with metastatic breast cancer and a 3-year history of zolendronate exposure. (B) Axial CT demonstrating the bony sequestrum (arrow) and extensive sclerosis of the left hemi-mandible. The patient had received oral and intravenous antibiotics with no improvement and presented with severe (10/10) pain not responsive to any type of narcotic therapy. (C) Bone scintigraphy with Tc99 demonstrates involvement of the left hemimandible. We elected to resect the left hemimandible transorally. (D) Intraoperative view of left hemimandible with bone sequestrum visible along the lingual aspect of the alveolar ridge. A custom bent osteosynthesis plate was placed. (E) Frontal view of patient 7 years postoperatively without recurrent MRONJ. (F) Intraoral view 7 years postoperatively. (G) Posteroanterior 3-dimensional (3D) image of the patient at 7 years status post left hemimandibulectomy with osteosynthesis reconstruction. (H) Lateral 3D image of patient 7 years status post left hemimandibulectomy with osteosynthesis reconstruction.

to be the indicated, treatment the following principles should be applied:

1. Appropriate preoperative imaging to assess the extent of disease,
2. Removal of all necrotic bone and any involved teeth to achieve disease-free bony margins,
3. Removal of any sharp bony edges and spicules,
4. Achievement of a layered tension-free primary wound closure whenever possible,
5. Culture-directed postoperative antibiotic therapy until mucosal healing is seen, and

6. Restraint from wearing any oral prosthetic devices until complete mucosal healing is seen.

Patients with stage 3 MRONJ who present with extensive maxillofacial involvement may benefit from wide local debridement or segmental resection of necrotic bone. We reserve this treatment for those with severe symptomatic disease when other modalities have failed. Segmental resection for treatment of stage 3 osteonecrosis of the jaw has shown generally favorable outcomes with up to a 90% success rate.[10,34,51,52] As with stage 2 disease, evidence of osteomyelitis at one of the

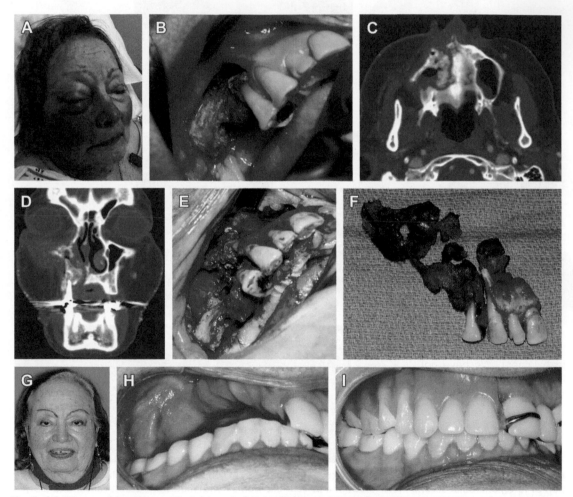

Fig. 4. (*A*) 74-year-old woman with right periorbital cellulitis and stage 3 maxillary medication-related osteonecrosis of the jaw (MRONJ). Her history was significant for multiple myeloma and 4 years of intravenous bisphosphonate therapy. Two years before admission, she had undergone extraction of the right maxillary second molar tooth, which failed to heal. She had been off and on oral antibiotic therapy since that time. (*B*) Intraoral view of exposed necrotic bone in the right maxilla. (*C*) Axial and (*D*) coronal CT demonstrating extensive MRONJ of the right hemimaxilla, right inferior turbinate, and orbital floor. (*E*) Right maxillary stage 3 MRONJ showing extent of necrosis. (*F*) Fragments of necrotic right maxilla, dentoalveolar bone, and associated dentition. (*G*) Frontal view 5 years postoperatively. She has had no recurrence of MRONJ. (*H*) Intraoral view without and (*I*) with prosthesis 5 years postoperatively.

resected margins is a predictor for recurrent disease.[34] Our experience with segmental resection in cases involving both the maxilla and mandible has overall been positive with successful long term resolution of MRONJ without recurrence. The same treatment principles outlined for stage 2 MRONJ also apply to patients with stage 3 disease.

Mandibular Resection

Once the decision to perform segmental mandibular resection is made, planning in our institution involves fine cut CT scanning for fabrication of a custom titanium osteosynthesis plate. The CT scan is also used to determine the extent of disease with a view toward identifying margins of viable bone. Depending on the patient's medical status, reconstruction may be limited to the osteosynthesis plate or may include microsurgical free tissue transfer. Double-layer primary closure of the wound margins is achieved, including primary closure of extraction sites in the surgical area. When reconstruction involves only the osteosynthesis plate we approach this transorally and have found we can perform a hemimandibulectomy with this method. The case presented in **Fig. 3** illustrates this approach.

Maxilla Resection

The same principles apply for treatment of stage 3 MRONJ involving the maxilla. All loose necrotic bone sequestra are removed and the area thoroughly debrided and when possible primary wound closure is performed. The majority of our cases have involved the posterior maxilla and we have seen unilateral and bilateral disease. CT is important to help delineate the extent of bony involvement. We have not used fluorescence to identify bony margins and have relied on preoperative imaging and the clinical appearance of the bone at the time of surgery. We have only used prosthetic appliances for maxillary reconstruction (**Fig. 4**). We have had no recurrences with our stage 3 cases to date.

SUMMARY

Treatment of MRONJ presents a challenging clinical dilemma. Based on current evidence, the best treatment is that which achieves the patient's goals and provides the best quality of life. In our experience, use of topical and oral antimicrobials, pentoxifylline, and vitamin E, with or without surgery leads to satisfactory outcomes.

REFERENCES

1. Ruggiero SL, Mehrotra B, Rosenberg TJ, et al. Osteonecrosis of the jaws associated with the use of bisphosphonates: a review of 63 cases. J Oral Maxillofac Surg 2004;62(5):527–34.
2. Kyrgidis A, Toulis KA. Denosumab-related osteonecrosis of the jaws. Osteoporos Int 2011;22(1):369–70.
3. Ruggiero SL, Dodson TB, Fantasia J, et al. American Association of Oral and Maxillofacial Surgeons position paper on medication-related osteonecrosis of the jaw–2014 update. J Oral Maxillofac Surg 2014; 72(10):1938–56.
4. Jenkins S, Addy M, Wade W, et al. The magnitude and duration of the effects of some mouthrinse products on salivary bacterial counts. J Clin Periodontol 1994;21(6):397–401.
5. Jenkins S, Addy M, Wade W. The mechanism of action of chlorhexidine. A study of plaque growth on enamel inserts in vivo. J Clin Periodontol 1988;15(7):415–24.
6. Gaffar A, Afflitto J, Nabi N. Chemical agents for the control of plaque and plaque microflora: an overview. Eur J Oral Sci 1997;105(5 Pt 2):502–7.
7. Moretti F, Pelliccioni GA, Montebugnoli L, et al. A prospective clinical trial for assessing the efficacy of a minimally invasive protocol in patients with bisphosphonate-associated osteonecrosis of the jaws. Oral Surg Oral Med Oral Pathol Oral Radiol Endod 2011;112(6):777–82.
8. Kumar SK, Gorur A, Schaudinn C, et al. The role of microbial biofilms in osteonecrosis of the jaw associated with bisphosphonatetherapy. Curr Osteoporos Rep 2010;8(1):40–8.
9. Ferlito S, Puzzo S, Palermo F, et al. Treatment of bisphosphonate-related osteonecrosis of the jaws: presentation of a protocol and an observational longitudinal study of an Italian series of cases. Br J Oral Maxillofac Surg 2012;50(5):425–9.
10. Rupel K, Ottaviani G, Gobbo M, et al. A systematic review of therapeutical approaches in bisphosphonates-related osteonecrosis of the jaw (BRONJ). Oral Oncol 2014;50(11):1049–57.
11. Hansen T, Kunkel M, Springer E, et al. Actinomycosis of the jaws—histopathological study of 45 patients shows significant involvement in bisphosphonate-associated osteonecrosis and infected osteoradionecrosis. Virchows Arch 2007;451:1009–17.
12. Sedghizadeh PP, Kumar SK, Gorur A, et al. Identification of microbial biofilms in osteonecrosis of the jaws secondary to bisphosphonate therapy. J Oral Maxillofac Surg 2008;66:767–75.
13. Pushalkar S, Li X, Kurago Z, et al. Oral microbiota and host innate immune response in bisphosphonate-related osteonecrosis of the jaw. Int J Oral Sci 2014; 6(4):219–26.
14. Wei X, Pushalkar S, Estilo C, et al. Molecular profiling of oral microbiota in jawbone samples of

bisphosphonate-related osteonecrosis of the jaw. Oral Dis 2012;18(6):602–12.

15. Hinson AM, Smith CW, Siegel ER, et al. Is bisphosphonate-related osteonecrosis of the jaw an infection? A histological and microbiological ten-year summary. Int J Dent 2014;2014:452737.

16. Wilson M. Susceptibility of oral bacterial biofilms to antimicrobial agents. J Med Microbiol 1996;44(2): 79–87.

17. Wu H, Moser C, Wang HZ, et al. Strategies for combating bacterial biofilm infections. Int J Oral Sci 2014;7(1):1–7.

18. Robard L, Louis MY, Blanchard D, et al. Medical treatment of osteoradionecrosis of the mandible by PENTOCLO: preliminary results. Eur Ann Otorhinolaryngol Head Neck Dis 2014;131(6):333–8.

19. Lyons A, Ghazali N. Osteoradionecrosis of the jaws: current understanding of its pathophysiology and treatment. Br J Oral Maxillofac Surg 2008;46(8): 653–60.

20. Delanian S, Chatel C, Porcher R, et al. Complete restoration of refractory mandibular osteoradionecrosis by prolonged treatment with apentoxifyllinetocopherol-clodronate combination (PENTOCLO): a phase II trial. Int J Radiat Oncol Biol Phys 2011; 80(3):832–9.

21. Epstein MS, Wicknick FW, Epstein JB, et al. Management of bisphosphonate-associated osteonecrosis: pentoxifylline and tocopherol in addition to antimicrobial therapy. An initial case series. Oral Surg Oral Med Oral Pathol Oral Radiol Endod 2010;110(5):593–6.

22. Brennan S, Salib O, O'Shea C, et al. A randomized prospective study of extended tocopherol and pentoxifylline therapy, in addition to carbogen, in the treatment of radiation late effects. Ecancermedicalscience 2008;2:81.

23. Ward A, Clissold SP. Pentoxifylline. A review of its pharmacodynamic and pharmacokinetic properties, and its therapeutic efficacy. Drugs 1987; 34(1):50–97.

24. Delanian S, Porcher R, Rudant J, et al. Kinetics of response to long-term treatment combining pentoxifylline and tocopherol in patients with superficial radiation-induced fibrosis. J Clin Oncol 2005; 23(34):8570–9.

25. Harper RP, Fung E. Resolution of bisphosphonate-associated osteonecrosis of the mandible: possible application for intermittent low-dose parathyroid hormone [rhPTH(1-34)]. J Oral Maxillofac Surg 2007; 65(3):573–80.

26. Lau AN, Adachi JD. Resolution of osteonecrosis of the jaw after teriparatide [recombinant human PTH-(1-34)] therapy. J Rheumatol 2009;36(8):1835–7.

27. Subramanian G, Cohen HV, Quek SY. A model for the pathogenesis of bisphosphonate-associated osteonecrosis of the jaw and teriparatide's potential role in its resolution. Oral Surg Oral Med Oral Pathol Oral Radiol Endod 2011;112(6):744–53.

28. Ohbayashi Y, Miyake M, Sawai F, et al. Adjunct teriparatide therapy with monitoring of bone turnover markers and bone scintigraphy for bisphosphonate-related osteonecrosis of the jaw. Oral Surg Oral Med Oral Pathol Oral Radiol Endod 2013;115(4): e31–7.

29. Freiberger JJ. Utility of hyperbaric oxygen in treatment of bisphosphonate-related osteonecrosis of the jaws. J Oral Maxillofac Surg 2009;67(5 Suppl): 96–106.

30. Freiberger JJ, Padilla-Burgos R, McGraw T, et al. What is the role of hyperbaric oxygen in the management of bisphosphonate-related osteonecrosis of the jaw: a randomized controlled trial of hyperbaric oxygen as an adjunct to surgery and antibiotics. J Oral Maxillofac Surg 2012; 70(7):1573–83.

31. Markose G, Mackenzie FR, Currie WJ, et al. Bisphosphonate osteonecrosis: a protocol for surgical management. Br J Oral Maxillofac Surg 2009;47(4): 294–7.

32. Wilde F, Heufelder M, Winter K, et al. The role of surgical therapy in the management of intravenous bisphosphonates-related osteonecrosis of the jaw. Oral Surg Oral Med Oral Pathol Oral Radiol Endod 2011;111(2):153–63.

33. Heufelder MJ, Hendricks J, Remmerbach T, et al. Principles of oral surgery for prevention of bisphosphonate-related osteonecrosis of the jaw. Oral Surg Oral Med Oral Pathol Oral Radiol Endod 2014;117(6):e429–35.

34. Bedogni A, Saia G, Bettini G, et al. Long-term outcomes of surgical resection of the jaws in cancer patients with bisphosphonate-related osteonecrosis. Oral Oncol 2011;47(5):420–4.

35. Saia G, Blandamura S, Bettini G, et al. Occurrence of bisphosphonate-related osteonecrosis of the jaw after surgical tooth extraction. J Oral Maxillofac Surg 2010;68(4):797–804.

36. O'Ryan FS, Khoury S, Liao W, et al. Intravenous bisphosphonate-related osteonecrosis of the jaw: bone scintigraphy as an early indicator. J Oral Maxillofac Surg 2009;67(7):1363–72.

37. Stockmann P, Hinkmann FM, Lell MM, et al. Panoramic radiograph, computed tomography or magnetic resonance imaging. Which imaging technique should be preferred in bisphosphonate-associated osteonecrosis of the jaw? A prospective clinical study. Clin Oral Investig 2010;14(3):311–7.

38. Guggenberger R, Fischer DR, Metzler P, et al. Bisphosphonate-induced osteonecrosis of the jaw: comparison of disease extent on contrast-enhanced MR imaging, [18F] fluoride PET/CT, and conebeam CT imaging. AJNR Am J Neuroradiol 2013;34(6):1242–7.

39. Pautke C, Bauer F, Otto S, et al. Fluorescence-guided bone resection in bisphosphonate-related osteonecrosis of the jaws: first clinical results of a prospective pilot study. J Oral Maxillofac Surg 2011;69(1):84–91.

40. Pautke C, Bauer F, Tischer T, et al. Fluorescence-guided bone resection in bisphosphonate-associated osteonecrosis of the jaws. J Oral Maxillofac Surg 2009;67(3):471–6.

41. Fleisher KE, Doty S, Kottal S, et al. Tetracycline-guided debridement and cone beam computed tomography for the treatment of bisphosphonate-related osteonecrosis of the jaw: a technical note. J Oral Maxillofac Surg 2008;66(12):2646–53.

42. Otto S, Baumann S, Ehrenfeld M, et al. Successful surgical management of osteonecrosis of the jaw due to RANK-ligand inhibitor treatment using fluorescence guided bone resection. J Craniomaxillofac Surg 2013;41(7):694–8.

43. Ristow O, Pautke C. Auto-fluorescence of the bone and its use for delineation of bone necrosis. Int J Oral Maxillofac Surg 2014;43(11):1391–3.

44. Del Fabbro M, Gallesio G, Mozzati M. Autologous platelet concentrates for bisphosphonate-related osteonecrosis of the jaw treatment and prevention. A systematic review of the literature. Eur J Cancer 2015;51(1):62–74.

45. Curi MM, Cossolin GS, Koga DH, et al. Bisphosphonate-related osteonecrosis of the jaws–an initial case series report of treatment combining partial bone resection and autologous platelet-rich plasma. J Oral Maxillofac Surg 2011;69(9):2465–72.

46. Angiero F, Sannino C, Borloni R, et al. Osteonecrosis of the jaws caused by bisphosphonates: evaluation of a new therapeutic approach using the Er:YAG laser. Lasers Med Sci 2009;24(6):849–56.

47. Rugani P, Acham S, Truschnegg A, et al. Bisphosphonate-associated osteonecrosis of the jaws: surgical treatment with ErCrYSGG-laser. Case report. Oral Surg Oral Med Oral Pathol Oral Radiol Endod 2010;110(6):e1–6.

48. Vescovi P, Merigo E, Meleti M, et al. Surgical approach and laser applications in BRONJ osteoporotic and cancer patients. J Osteoporos 2012;2012:585434.

49. Vescovi P, Merigo E, Meleti M, et al. Bisphosphonates-related osteonecrosis of the jaws: a concise review of the literature and a report of a single-centre experience with 151 patients. J Oral Pathol Med 2012;41(3):214–21.

50. Vescovi P, Manfredi M, Merigo E, et al. Early surgical laser-assisted management of bisphosphonate-related osteonecrosis of the jaws (BRONJ): a retrospective analysis of 101 treated sites with long-term follow-up. Photomed Laser Surg 2012;30(1):5–13.

51. Carlson ER, Basile JD. The role of surgical resection in the management of bisphosphonate-related osteonecrosis of the jaws. J Oral Maxillofac Surg 2009;67(5 Suppl):85–95.

52. Graziani F, Vescovi P, Campisi G, et al. Resective surgical approach shows a high performance in the management of advanced cases of bisphosphonate-related osteonecrosis of the jaws: a retrospective survey of 347 cases. J Oral Maxillofac Surg 2012;70(11):2501–7.

Preventive Strategies for Patients at Risk of Medication-related Osteonecrosis of the Jaw

Reginald H. Goodday, DDS, MSc, FRCD(C), FICD, FACD

KEYWORDS

- Osteonecrosis of the jaw (ONJ) • Bisphosphonates • Antiresorptives • Risk • Prevention

KEY POINTS

- For patients at risk, information can be provided by the pharmaceutical manufacturer, pharmacist, prescribing physician, dentist, and oral and maxillofacial surgeon.
- Prevention strategies to reduce the incidence of osteonecrosis should be applied as soon as it is determined that a patient will be placed on antiresorptive medication.
- Proper screening involves a comprehensive oral examination with radiographs followed by oral hygiene instruction and necessary dental treatment; surgical techniques and adjunctive therapies that favor optimum healing of bone and soft tissue decrease the risk of osteonecrosis of the jaw.
- Because of the low incidence of osteonecrosis of the jaw, no dental procedures are absolutely contraindicated.
- The published evidence to date supports the following recommendations:

Comprehensive oral examination with appropriate radiographs

Oral hygiene instruction

Maintenance of good oral health

Completion of necessary dental treatment

Use of antibiotics before and after surgery

Use of antimicrobial mouth rinses

Drug holiday when indicated

INTRODUCTION

Oral and maxillofacial surgeons first recognized and reported cases of nonhealing exposed bone in the maxillofacial region of patients treated with intravenous (IV) bisphosphonates in 2003[1,2] (**Fig. 1**). Subsequently the same type of lesion was observed in patients taking oral bisphosphonate medication and recently other antiresorptive drugs and angiogenesis inhibitors. These lesions are now called medication-related osteonecrosis of the jaw (MRONJ).[3] Because of its recent observation and low incidence, this is a condition that is not well understood or well managed by many health care professionals. However, there are various levels of evidence that support different strategies that decrease the risk of osteonecrosis of the jaw (ONJ) (**Box 1**).

Various guides and recommendations exist on the prevention of ONJ; however, most information available to guide decision making has been derived from case series and retrospective

Department of Oral and Maxillofacial Sciences, Faculty of Dentistry, Dalhousie University, 5981 University Avenue, Halifax, Nova Scotia B3H 4R2, Canada
E-mail address: reginald.goodday@dal.ca

Oral Maxillofacial Surg Clin N Am 27 (2015) 527–536
http://dx.doi.org/10.1016/j.coms.2015.06.006
1042-3699/15/$ – see front matter

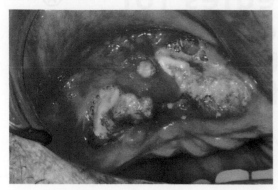

Fig. 1. Nonhealing exposed bone in the right maxilla of a 59-year-old patient with multiple myeloma treated with IV bisphosphonate therapy for 1 year. Patient history included the spontaneous exfoliation of an infected retained maxillary tooth root in the bicuspid region 2 months earlier.

Box 1
Strategies to prevent MRONJ

Patient awareness of risk
- Pharmaceutical manufacturer
- Pharmacist
- Prescribing physician
- Dentist
- Oral and maxillofacial surgeon

Dental screening
- Oral examination
- Radiographs
- Oral hygiene instruction
- Patient education

Treatment
- Surgery before initiation of medication therapy
- Elimination of inflammation/infection
- Fluoride application
- Prophylactic antibiotics before/after surgery
- Chlorhexidine rinses
- Drug holiday during healing phase
- Elimination of ill-fitting dentures

Potential risk-reducing modalities
- Plasma rich in growth factors
- Neodymium:yttrium-aluminum-garnet laser therapy
- Locally applied sodium bicarbonate
- Autologous platelet concentrate
- Parathyroid hormone therapy

---

observational and cohort studies. There has not been sufficient time to gather abundant evidence based on prospective randomized trials with adequate sample size to provide category 1 recommendations for the prevention of ONJ.

MRONJ is a painful, debilitating condition that is difficult to treat and even more difficult to cure. Benjamin Franklin's advice that an ounce of prevention is worth a pound of cure is particularly applicable to this condition.

Ideally, prevention strategies to reduce the incidence of MRONJ should be applied as soon as it is determined that a patient should be placed on antiresorptive medication. If this medication has already been initiated there are strategies that can still be considered by clinicians to decrease the risk of ONJ.

Prevention strategies involve multiple groups:

- Pharmaceutical manufacturers include this possible adverse event in the package insert of medication associated with ONJ. They advise that, "A dental examination with appropriate preventive dentistry should be considered prior to treatment with bisphosphonates."[4]
- Pharmacists can advise the patient of the risk of osteonecrosis and advocate the value of a consultation with a member of the dental profession in reducing this risk.
- Physicians prescribing antiresorptive or antiangiogenic medications should counsel patients on possible oral complications resulting from taking this medication and advise their patients to consult directly with a dentist or oral and maxillofacial surgeon. However, this does not seem to be happening. Migliorati and colleagues[5] recently conducted a single-center observational study involving 73 patients seeking routine dental care while taking bisphosphonates. Eighty-two percent said that they had not been told about the possible side effects of taking bisphosphonates. Participants reported having no knowledge of ONJ and reported that their physicians had not told them that they needed to inform their dentists that they were receiving bisphosphonate therapy.
- Dentists and oral and maxillofacial surgeons have a responsibility to be aware of the risks of antiresorptive medication and to be prepared to inform, educate, and treat these patients.
- Patients need to be compliant and follow the recommendations and instructions by their dentist/oral surgeon, especially those pertaining to the maintenance of good oral hygiene and use of antibiotics.

PATIENTS AT RISK

The first step in a preventive strategy is to identify those patients who are considered at risk. The incidence of ONJ seems to vary based on the medication that has been prescribed. In general, the duration of antiresorptive medication increases the risk of ONJ, with the incidence reaching a plateau after 2 to 4 years depending on the type of medication.[3]

To appreciate the effect of the drug on jaw necrosis, it is important to be aware that controlled studies with patients with cancer who were assigned to a placebo group have shown the risk of spontaneous ONJ to range between 0% and 0.019% or 0 to 1.9 cases per 10,000.[6–8] In patients with osteoporosis assigned to a placebo group the risk of spontaneous ONJ is 0% to 0.02% or 0 to 2 cases per 10,000 patients.[9,10]

Medication Related to Osteonecrosis of the Jaw

Bisphosphonates

Mechanism of action: inhibition of osteoclast bone resorption and remodeling to prevent bone fracture.

Indication: IV bisphosphonates are used to manage cancer-related conditions affecting bone metastasis from breast, prostate, lung, and bone lesions caused by multiple myeloma and osteoporosis.

Example: zoledronate (Zometa)

Incidence of ONJ: in patients with cancer, the risk is approximately 1% or 100 cases per 10,000.[6–8,11] This risk is 50 to 100 times higher than in patients treated with placebo.[3]

In patients with osteoporosis treated with IV bisphosphonate for 3 years the risk is 0.017% or 1.7 cases per 10,000.[10]

Indication: oral bisphosphonates are approved for the treatment of osteopenia and osteoporosis.

Example: alendronate (Fosamax)

Incidence of ONJ: in patients with osteoporosis using oral bisphosphonates the risk is 0.1% or 10 cases per 100,000, and for patients on oral bisphosphonates for greater than 4 years the incidence increases to 0.21% or 21 cases per 10,000.[12]

Receptor activator of nuclear factor kappa-B ligand inhibitor

Mechanism of action: a fully humanized monoclonal antibody that inhibits receptor activator of nuclear factor kappa-B ligand (RANKL)

protein, which acts as a signal for bone removal and decreases osteoclast function.

Indication: used in osteoporotic patients and patients with metastatic bone disease to prevent bone fracture.

Example: denosumab (Xgeva, Prolia)

Incidence of ONJ: in patients with cancer treated with a RANKL inhibitor the risk of ONJ is approximately 0.8% or 80 cases per 10,000 patients.[6,9]

Angiogenesis inhibitors

Mechanism of action: interfere with the formation of new blood vessels and have shown efficacy in the treatment of several malignancies.

Indication: treatment of gastrointestinal tumors, renal cell carcinoma, neuroendocrine tumors, and other malignancies.

Example: bevacizumab (Avastin)

Incidence of ONJ: in patients with cancer the risk is 0.2% or 20 cases per 100,000.[13]

PREVENTIVE STRATEGIES BEFORE COMMENCEMENT OF ANTIRESORPTIVES
Dental Screening

For prevention of MRONJ, the most common recommendation worldwide is to complete necessary oral surgery before initiation of antiresorptive medication and when possible avoid dental extractions after this medication is started. This avoidance strategy identifies the importance of appropriate screening by the dental profession when it is apparent that the patient would benefit from taking antiresorptive medication. A multidisciplinary approach to these patients includes consultation with the appropriate dental professional. Early screening and initiation of appropriate dental care not only decreases the incidence of ONJ but also provides all patients with the benefits of optimum oral health.

Ripamonti and colleagues[14] conducted the first study to compare a prospective group in a dental prevention program with a retrospective group that did not undergo any dental preventive measure. They used a retrospective group for comparison because, in their opinion, it would not be ethical to conduct a controlled study in which patients are randomized such that one group would be denied preventive dental measures. Their article concluded that there is an important reduction in the incidence of ONJ in those patients who received appropriate dental prevention measures compared with the group that did not. In their opinion, the identification of patients at risk combined with a dental examination can improve outcomes and increase the number of ONJ-free patients. They recommended screening and providing appropriate dental preventive measures before initiating drug therapy.[14]

Dimopoulos and colleagues[15] published a similar study that investigated whether the incidence of ONJ in 90 consecutive patients decreased after the implementation of preventive measures compared with 38 patients who received the drug before dental screening. There was a statistically significant, almost 3-fold reduction in the incidence of osteonecrosis in patients when preventive measures were applied. These measures included all patients being screened by a dentist, with all dental work completed before the start of drug therapy, and all patients were advised to maintain good oral hygiene.

Bonacina and colleagues[16] evaluated the effectiveness of oral and dental prevention strategies for patients with cancer who were about to begin IV bisphosphonate therapy. Two hundred and eighty-two consecutive patients planned for drug therapy were screened in a dental department. Two-hundred and seventeen patients received necessary dental treatment before initiating IV bisphosphonate treatment. The other 65 patients who had received previous bisphosphonate therapy and for whom dental risk factors were identified were informed of the possible risk of ONJ. The necessary oral and hygiene restorative and rehabilitation therapy was offered to these patients. The 2 groups were compared and all new cases of ONJ developed in patients who previously underwent therapy with bisphosphonates. The investigators support the implementation of dental screening before initiating drug therapy and a preventive regime that involves the maintenance of good oral hygiene during therapy.

A prospective single-center study conducted by Vandone and colleagues[17] in 2012 assessed the efficacy of a preventive, restorative dental care program in the reduction of ONJ risk. It compared a prospective group of 211 patients who underwent preventive dental care with a retrospective group of 200 patients who did not. The incidence rate of developing ONJ was half in the patients who were screened and received preventive care. It is the investigators' opinion that patients unable to undertake preventive dental measures before bisphosphonate treatment still benefit from reaching and maintaining a stable oral condition during therapy because good oral health seems to minimize the risk of developing ONJ.[17]

In the same year, Saad and colleagues[18] published a multicenter prospective trial involving 5723 patients, assessing ONJ incidence, risk factors, and outcomes in patients receiving bisphosphonates for metastatic bone disease. Tooth extraction (61.8%) was the predominant oral factor associated with the development of ONJ (1.6% of all patients). In the investigators' opinion, this finding emphasized the importance of assessing oral health in patients and implementing the required preventive dentistry before initiating therapy. Their conclusions were that "ONJ was infrequent, management was mostly conservative, and healing occurred in over one-third of the patients. Educating physicians about oral health before and during bone-targeted therapy may help reduce ONJ incidence and improve outcomes."[18] The investigators stated that, "This finding emphasizes the importance of assessing oral health of patients and implementing preventive dentistry if necessary before initiating therapy". "Once antiresorptive therapy has been initiated, the aim should be maintenance of good oral health and avoidance of elective extractions."[18]

In 2013, Wong and colleagues[19] reviewed the available evidence pertaining to ONJ resulting from medical treatment of nonmalignant bone disease. This article points out that published guidelines regarding prevention and treatment of ONJ exist, but they are based on expert opinion rather than firm data. In the investigators' opinion it is sensible to arrange dental review before bisphosphonate commencement so that any invasive dental procedures can be performed beforehand.

Hinchy and colleagues[20] considered that the theory behind preradiation assessments holds true before chemotherapy in that prechemotherapy comprehensive oral evaluations are an attempt to anticipate as well as prevent ONJ. All patients newly diagnosed with multiple myeloma or oncologic disease that has metastasized should be offered a comprehensive dental evaluation. Treatment planning needs to eliminate both acute infections and areas of potential infection to prevent future sequelae that could be exacerbated once drug therapies begin. Consideration includes patients' motivation, infection, fluoride applications, chlorhexidine rinses, patient education regarding dental care, and elimination of all possible local contributors to ONJ before initiation of drug therapy.[20]

Most recently, Bramati and colleagues[21] investigated the occurrence of ONJ after implementation of dental preventive measures before starting and during bisphosphonate therapy. In this prospective study with a 6-year follow-up, of 212 patients treated with bisphosphonates for bone metastasis, no case of ONJ was recorded. It is the investigators' opinion that a strict preventive program can prevent ONJ.

The significant reduction in the incidence of ONJ as reported in these studies supports the important role of screening by dental professionals as a preventive strategy in the reduction of risk of antiresorptive agent–induced ONJ. Proper screening involves a comprehensive oral examination with radiographs followed by oral hygiene instruction and necessary dental treatment.

PREVENTIVE STRATEGIES AFTER COMMENCEMENT OF ANTIRESORPTIVES
Dentoalveolar Surgery

Dentoalveolar surgery is the major risk factor for ONJ. A history of a tooth extraction is found in 52% to 61% of patients with ONJ.[18,22,23] When root resection and cystectomy are included, the incidence is 80%.[24] The estimates for developing ONJ after tooth extraction in patients with cancer exposed to IV bisphosphonates ranges from 1.6% to 14.8%.[3] The best estimate for risk of ONJ in patients exposed to oral bisphosphonates after tooth extraction is 0.5%.[25]

Despite the evidence of the risk of surgery in patients treated with antiresorptive medication, the necessity to perform surgery does arise. Following protocols that can reduce the incidence of MRONJ is therefore very important, but level 1 evidence–based guidelines for the management of dental extractions in these patients is deficient. However, surgical techniques and adjunctive therapies that favor optimum healing of bone and soft tissue decrease the risk of ONJ.

Recent research has suggested the possibility that bisphosphonates could increase bacterial colonization and biofilm formation in patients treated with these drugs. This possibility would explain some unclear aspects of the pathophysiology of bisphosphonate-related ONJ, including the prevalent appearance after bone exposure and the recurrent nature of osteomyelitis accompanying the use of this medication. Exposure of bone during dental surgery acts as a trigger for bacterial invasion. The presence of bisphosphonates promotes bacterial adhesion and biofilm formation on the surface of the affected bone, which is an essential step in the development of persistent osteomyelitis. It would justify antimicrobial treatment in MRONJ. The critical role of bacterial infection in the pathogenesis of MRONJ is also supported by clinical data showing that improvement of dental hygiene decreases the incidence of bisphosphonate-related ONJ in patients with multiple myeloma and metastatic cancer.[26]

When extraction or bone surgery is required, the use of a chlorhexidine rinse is recommended before surgery and on a twice to 3 times daily basis until the surgical site has healed.[24,27,28]

Several investigators recommend the use of prophylactic antibiotics when extracting teeth in patients on antiresorptive medication. Montefusco and colleagues[28] reviewed patients with multiple myeloma treated with bisphosphonate receiving dental procedures. Out of 114 patients, there were 8 cases of ONJ in the 71 patients who did not receive prophylactic antibiotics. There were no cases of ONJ in 43 patients with prophylaxis.[28]

In a recent prospective study, Heufelder and colleagues[24] evaluated treatment procedures to establish surgical methods for prevention of bisphosphonate ONJ for patients at risk because of present or previous bisphosphonate therapy. Their protocol included preoperative oral antibiotics for 7 days, starting 48 hours before surgical intervention. All patients received amoxicillin and clavulanic acid (875 mg/125 mg) every 12 hours or, in cases of penicillin allergy, clindamycin (600 mg) every 8 hours. Out of 117 surgical procedures performed in 68 patients, only 3 patients with a long history of IV bisphosphonate medication developed MRONJ 4 weeks after surgery. Two of the 3 cases developed in patients with former MRONJ.[24]

Several investigators have suggested the need to raise a full mucoperiosteal flap to achieve primary closure after a simple extraction. However, Mozzati and colleagues[29] showed that there is no need to have primary closure of the socket in a prospective study of 700 consecutive patients treated with oral bisphosphonates with no evidence of postoperative ONJ. All patients received a professional oral hygiene session 1 week before surgery and were given 1 tablet of amoxicillin and clavulanic acid twice a day for a total of 6 days starting the evening before the surgery. Patients allergic to penicillin were given erythromycin. One group had surgical extraction with full-thickness flaps to allow wound healing via primary intention. In the second group, the sockets were filled with absorbable gelatin sponge hemostatic to allow wound healing via secondary intention. No intraoperative complications were found in either group.[29]

Forced eruption as an alternative to tooth extraction in long-term use of oral bisphosphonates has been recommended by Smidt and colleagues[30] as an option when a patient refuses to undergo conventional tooth extraction. The combination of orthodontic extrusion and bloodless extraction is designed to minimize trauma and enhance the health of the surrounding tissues.

New Risk-reducing Strategies at Time of Extraction

In a prospective study, Scoletta and colleagues[31] evaluated 63 patients with a history of IV bisphosphonate treatment and requiring dental surgery. They observed that filling the extraction sites with autologous plasma rich in growth factors (PRGF) eliminates the need for primary closure using a vestibular flap. These results support the findings of an earlier case control study by Mozzati and colleagues[32] that assessed the use of PRGF in patients on IV bisphosphonates and requiring tooth extraction. In the 91 patients treated with PRGF there were no cases of ONJ, compared with 5 cases of ONJ in the control group of 85 patients not treated with PRGF.[32]

Vescovi and colleagues[33] reported on the usefulness of oral hygiene, prophylactic antibiotics, mouth rinses, and neodymium:yttrium-aluminum-garnet laser therapy in the surgical management of patients on oral and IV bisphosphonates. Their case series reviewed the healing of 589 tooth extractions in 217 patients. One week before dental extraction professional oral hygiene procedures were performed. Amoxicillin 2 g/d were administered 3 days before and for 2 weeks after tooth extraction and suture removal. After extraction, the sockets were irrigated with povidone-iodine. Mouthwashes with chlorhexidine 3 times per day were recommended until complete mucosal healing. Patients received a low-level laser therapy delivered in the postextraction socket once a week for 6 weeks. Complete healing occurred, except for minimal bone exposure that was observed after 5 tooth extractions in 5 patients with cancer out of a total of 589 extractions for an incidence of 0.85%. The investigators concluded that the combination of antibiotic treatment, the suggested prophylactic protocol, and low-level laser therapy has been effective for reducing the incidence of MRONJ after tooth extractions in patients already debilitated by systemic disease.[33]

Dayisoylu and colleagues[34] investigated the preventive effects of locally applied sodium bicarbonate on bisphosphonate-related ONJ in an animal model. No ONJ was observed in the animals receiving sodium bicarbonate. It was thought that locally applied sodium bicarbonate could compensate for the sudden decline in medium PH after tooth extraction or other invasive dental procedures. This locally increased alkaline phosphatase activity and the phagocytosis of macrophage-derived cells without toxicity might yield significant improvement in the preventive therapy and could be provided before the onset of MRONJ. Therefore alternative strategies, such as the use of alkalizing oral mouth rinses or alkaline pastes, may be helpful for the prevention of MRONJ. In this pilot study the results of the animal model were promising and require further investigation.

Del Fabbro and colleagues[35] conducted a systematic review of the literature designed to evaluate whether autologous platelet concentrates (APC) may improve treatment and prevention of MRONJ in patients under bisphosphonate therapy. Their review of 18 studies found that APC was associated with a lower MRONJ incidence after tooth extraction, although this was not significant. They concluded that their results should be cautiously interpreted because of the low evidence level of the studies included and the limited sample size. However, the results are suggestive of possible benefits of APC when associated with surgical procedures for treatment or prevention of MRONJ. To confirm such indications prospective comparative studies with a large sample size are urgently needed.

Kuroshima and colleagues[36] reported on 2 animal studies of the effect of parathyroid hormone (PTH) therapy on healing of tooth extraction sites. PTH therapy accelerated the entire healing process and promoted both hard and soft tissue healing by increasing bone fill and soft tissue maturation. PTH therapy by intraoral injection was as effective as subcutaneous injection in promoting tooth extraction socket healing. Further research may confirm the utility of this therapy in preventing ONJ in patients on antiresorptive medication.[36]

Implants

The literature is not clear on the risk of ONJ after implant surgery. The recent American Association of Oral and Maxillofacial Surgeons position paper on MRONJ recommends avoiding the placement of dental implants in oncologic patients receiving IV antiresorptive therapy or antiangiogenic medications. However, this paper also says that, in light of absent data, the risk for ONJ after dental implant placement requires exposure and manipulation of bone to be comparable with the risk associated with tooth extraction.[3]

The American Dental Association (ADA) advisory committee on antiresorptive therapy is of the opinion that the lack of reports associating ONJ with the placement of implants is encouraging and recommends that dentists inform patients that the risk of developing ONJ is low and the success rate seems to be no different than in patients without a history of bisphosphonate treatment. Note that this committee acknowledges the need for large, long-term studies to determine whether implants placed in patients exposed to antiresorptive agents perform as well as those placed in patients not exposed to these agents.[37]

Endodontics

In patients with an increased risk of developing MRONJ, endodontic treatment is preferable to surgical manipulation if a tooth is salvageable. The ADA advisory committee recommends that practitioners should use a routine endodontic technique, but manipulation should not take place beyond the tooth apex. Limited evidence shows that periapical healing after endodontic therapy is similar regardless of whether or not the patient has a history of bisphosphonate use. Endodontic surgical procedures should be guided by the same recommendation as used for oral and maxillofacial surgical procedures.[37]

Periodontics

Periodontitis occurs in 71% to 84% of ONJ cases, suggesting that it may be a risk factor.[38–40] Tsao and colleagues[41] conducted a cross-sectional study comparing cancer patients with an ONJ history following treatment with IV bisphosphonates with controls. This research showed an association of periodontitis with ONJ. The results suggest that the role of periodontitis-associated microbes as a contributing causal agent may have been overestimated.[41]

The ADA advisory committee recommends that patients receiving antiresorptive therapy who have active chronic periodontal disease generally should receive appropriate forms of nonsurgical therapy combined with a reevaluation of 4 to 6 weeks. There are no published studies in which investigators have evaluated the risk of MRONJ after periodontal procedures such as guided tissue regeneration or bone grafting. Use of such techniques should be considered judiciously from the patient's need. Primary soft tissue closure after periodontal surgical procedures is desirable, when feasible, although extended periodontal bone exposure for the sake of primary closure may increase, rather than decrease, the risk of developing MRONJ. Patients who do not have periodontal disease should receive preventive therapy or instruction in prevention of periodontal disease.[37] Periodontal surgical procedures should follow the same guidelines as oral and maxillofacial procedures.

Drug Holiday

Because the greatest risk of ONJ is from treatment with IV bisphosphonates, it is reasonable to think that to discontinue this medication before surgery would be a risk-reducing strategy. However, bisphosphonates are unique in that they bind to bone and are internalized by osteoclasts and remain in bone for years. Although there have been recommendations to discontinue this medication for 2 to 3 months before surgery there is lack of evidence confirming the value of doing so. Discontinuing the bisphosphonate most likely does not result in a drug holiday because persistence of the antiresorptive effect is expected for an undefined lengthy period of time.

This unique property of bisphosphonates makes it difficult to control this unwanted side effect and underscores the importance of optimizing dental health before initiating antiresorptive therapy whenever possible.

The International Task Force on Osteonecrosis of the Jaw does not recommend a drug holiday before surgery. They suggest that, "in those patients at high risk for the development of ONJ, including cancer patients receiving high dose BP [bisphosphonates] or DMAB [denosumab] therapy, consideration should be given to withholding antiresorptive therapy following extensive oral surgery until the surgical site heals with mature mucosal coverage." This task force suggests a drug holiday for approximately 6 weeks starting at the time of surgery because it eliminates active uptake of the drug by healing bone after surgery. This recommendation does not pertain to patients on oral bisphosphonates because they think that the antiresorptive medication does not need to be discontinued.[42]

The ADA considers that, because discontinuation of bisphosphonate therapy may not eliminate the risk of developing ONJ, there needs to be significant dental risks present to consider doing so.[37]

McClung and colleagues[43] are of the opinion that patients receiving bisphosphonates who are not at high risk for fracture are potential candidates for a drug holiday, whereas, in those with bone mineral density in the osteoporotic range or previous history of fragility fracture, the benefits of continuing therapy probably far outweigh the risk of harm.[43]

Damm and Jones[44] recently published an article with suggestions for a pattern of patient care for individuals receiving antiresorptive therapy who desire or require an invasive surgical procedure of the jaws but who also have a skeleton that is at risk for osteoporotic fracture. Based on bone physiology and pharmacokinetics, they recommend modification of the antiresorptive therapy and timing of the oral surgical procedure that minimize the prevalence of osteonecrosis while at the same time continuing to protect the patient's skeleton from osteoporotic fracture. In their opinion, because free bisphosphonate within the serum is usually at extremely low levels 2 months after the last dose of an oral bisphosphonate, a 2-month drug-free period should be adequate before an invasive dental procedure.[44] This modified drug holiday for osteoporotic patients is supported in the recent 2014 update of the American Association of Oral and Maxillofacial surgeons' position paper on MRONJ.[3]

If there is consideration of a drug holiday, it is important to discuss the risks and benefits of doing so with the prescribing physician.

SUMMARY

Patients receiving antiresorptive therapy who may require invasive surgical procedures should be informed that there is the risk, albeit small, of developing MRONJ. However, if it does occur, it can be painful, debilitating, and disconcerting to the patient. For those at risk, patient information can be provided by the pharmaceutical manufacturer, pharmacist, prescribing physician, dentist, and oral and maxillofacial surgeon. Through the education process, patients need to be advised of their responsibility in being compliant in maintaining good oral health.

The unique properties of the most commonly used antiresorptive medication are such that the resulting jaw lesions are difficult to cure, which means that the best strategies to prevent MRONJ are those completed before the initiation of antiresorptive therapy.

The published evidence to date supports the following recommendations:

- Comprehensive oral examination with appropriate radiographs
- Oral hygiene instruction
- Maintenance of good oral health
- Completion of necessary dental treatment
- Use of antibiotics before and after surgery
- Use of antimicrobial mouth rinses
- Drug holiday when indicated

Because of the low incidence of ONJ, no dental procedures are absolutely contraindicated. However, it is important for patients to be aware of the risk of ONJ based on the medication prescribed, how these lesions will affect their quality of life (pain, function, and so forth) and what measures they can take that have a favorable influence on preventing ONJ.

REFERENCES

1. Marx RE. Pamidronate (Aredia) and zoledronate (Xometa) induced avascular necrosis of the jaws: a growing epidemic. J Oral Maxillofac Surg 2003;61: 1115.
2. Ruggiero S, Mehrotra B, Rosenberg TJ, et al. Osteonecrosis of the jaws associated with the use of bisphosphonates: a review of 63 cases. J Oral Maxillofac Surg 2004;62:527–34.
3. Ruggiero S, Dodson T, Fantasia J, et al. American Association of oral and maxillofacial surgeons position paper on medication-related osteonecrosis of the jaw–2014 update. J Oral Maxillofac Surg 2014; 72:1938–56.
4. Product monograph, Fosamax. Bone metabolism regulator. Kirkland, Quebec: Merck Canada Inc. 2013;1–41.
5. Migliorati C, Mattos K, Palazzolo M. How patients' lack of knowledge about oral bisphosphonates can interfere with medical and dental care. J Am Dent Assoc 2010;141(5):562–6.
6. Qi W, Tang L, He A, et al. Risk of osteonecrosis of the jaw in cancer patients receiving denosumab: a meta-analysis of seven randomized controlled trials. Int J Clin Oncol 2014;19:403–10.
7. Coleman R, Woodward E, Brown J, et al. Safety of zoledronic acid and incidence of osteonecrosis of the jaw (ONJ) during adjuvant therapy in a randomised phase III trial (AZURE: BIG 01-04) for women with stage II/III breast cancer. Breast Cancer Res Treat 2011;127:429–38.
8. Mauri D, Valachis A, Polyzos I, et al. Osteonecrosis of the jaw and use of bisphosphonates in adjuvant breast cancer treatment: a meta-analysis. Breast Cancer Res Treat 2009;116:433–9.
9. Papapoulos S, Chapurlat R, Libanati C, et al. Five years of denosumab exposure in women with postmenopausal osteoporosis: results from the first two years of the FREEDOM extension. J Bone Miner Res 2012;27(3):694–701.
10. Grbic J, Black D, Lyles K, et al. The incidence of osteonecrosis of the jaw in patients receiving 5 milligrams of zoledronic acid: data from the health outcomes and reduced incidence with zoledronic acid once yearly clinical trials program. J Am Dent Assoc 2010;141:1365–70.
11. Scagliotti G, Hirsh V, Siena S, et al. Overall survival improvement in patients with lung cancer and bone metastases treated with denosumab versus zoledronic acid: subgroup analysis from a randomized phase 3 study. J Thorac Oncol 2012;7:1823–9.
12. Lo J, O'Ryan F, Gordon N, et al. Prevalence of osteonecrosis of the jaw in patients with oral bisphosphonate exposure. J Oral Maxillofac Surg 2010;68:243–53.
13. Guarneri V, Miles D, Robert N, et al. Bevacizumab and osteonecrosis of the jaw: incidence and association with bisphosphonate therapy in three large prospective trials in advanced breast cancer. Breast Cancer Res Treat 2010;122:181–8.
14. Ripamonti C, Maniezzo M, Campa T, et al. Decreased occurrence of osteonecrosis of the jaw

after implementation of dental preventive measures in solid tumour patients with bone metastases treated with bisphosphonates. The experience of the National Cancer Institute of Milan. Ann Oncol 2009;20(1):137–45.

15. Dimopoulos M, Kastritis E, Bamia C, et al. Reduction of osteonecrosis of the jaw (ONJ) after implementation of preventive measures in patients with multiple myeloma treated with zoledronic acid. Ann Oncol 2009;20(1):117–20.

16. Bonacina R, Mariani U, Villa F, et al. Preventive strategies and clinical implications for bisphosphonate-related osteonecrosis of the jaw: a review of 282 patients. J Can Dent Assoc 2011;77:B147.

17. Vandone A, Donadio M, Mozzati M, et al. Impact of dental care in the prevention of bisphosphonate-associated osteonecrosis of the jaw: a single-center clinical experience. Ann Oncol 2012;23(1):193–200.

18. Saad F, Brown JE, Van Poznak C, et al. Incidence, risk factors, and outcomes of osteonecrosis of the jaw: integrated analysis from three blinded active-controlled phase III trials in cancer patients with bone metastases. Ann Oncol 2012;23(5):1341–7.

19. Wong P, Borromeo G, Wark J. Bisphosphonate-related osteonecrosis of the jaw in non-malignant bone disease. Rheumatol Int 2013;33:2189–98.

20. Hinchy NV, Jayaprakash V, Rossitto RA, et al. Osteonecrosis of the jaw – Prevention and treatment strategies for oral health professionals. Oral Oncol 2013; 49:878–86.

21. Bramati A, Girelli S, Farina G, et al. Prospective, mono-institutional study of the impact of a systematic prevention program on incidence and outcome of osteonecrosis of the jaw in patients treated with bisphosphonates for bone metastases. J Bone Miner Metab 2015;33(1):119–24.

22. Vahtsevanos K, Kyrgidis A, Verrou E, et al. Longitudinal cohort study of risk factors in cancer patients of bisphosphonate-related osteonecrosis of the jaw. J Clin Oncol 2009;27:5356–62.

23. Fehm T, Beck V, Banys M, et al. Bisphosphonate-induced osteonecrosis of the jaw (ONJ): Incidence and risk factors in patients with breast cancer and gynecological malignancies. Gynecol Oncol 2009; 112:605–9.

24. Heufelder MJ, Hendricks J, Remmerbach T, et al. Principles of oral surgery for prevention of bisphosphonate-related osteonecrosis of the jaw. Oral Surg Oral Med Oral Pathol Oral Radiol 2014; 117:e429–435.

25. Kunchur R, Need A, Hughes T, et al. Clinical investigation of C-terminal cross-linking telopeptide test in prevention and management of bisphosphonate-associated osteonecrosis of the jaws. J Oral Maxillofac Surg 2009;67:1167–73.

26. Kos M, Junka A, Smutnicka D, et al. Pamidronate enhances bacterial adhesion to bone hydroxyapatite.

Another puzzle in the pathology of bisphosphonate-related osteonecrosis of the jaw? J Oral Maxillofac Surg 2013;71:1010–6.

27. Lodi G, Sardella A, Salis A, et al. Tooth extraction in patients taking intravenous bisphosphonates preventive protocol and case series. J Oral Maxillofac Surg 2010;68(1):107–10.

28. Montefusco V, Gay F, Spina F, et al. Antibiotic prophylaxis before dental procedures may reduce the incidence of osteonecrosis of the jaw in patients with multiple myeloma treated with bisphosphonates. Leuk Lymphoma 2008;49(11):2156–62.

29. Mozzati M, Arata V, Gallesio G. Tooth extractions in osteoporotic patients taking oral bisphosphonates. Osteoporos Int 2013;24:1707–12.

30. Smidt A, Lipovestsy-Adler M, Sharon E. Forced eruption as an alternative to tooth extraction in long-term use of oral bisphosphonates. J Am Dent Assoc 2012;143(12):1303–12.

31. Scoletta M, Arata V, Arduino P, et al. Tooth extractions in intravenous bisphosphonate-treated patient: a refined protocol. J Oral Maxillofac Surg 2013;71: 994–9.

32. Mozzati M, Arata V, Gallesio G. Tooth extraction in patients on zoledronic acid therapy. Oral Oncol 2012;48:817–21.

33. Vescovi P, Meleti M, Merigo E, et al. Case series of 589 extractions in patients under bisphosphonates therapy. Proposal of a clinical protocol supported by Nd:YAG low-level laser therapy. Med Oral Patol Oral Cir Bucal 2013;18(4):e680–5.

34. Dayisoylu E, Ungor C, Tosun E, et al. Does an alkaline environment prevent the development of bisphosphonate-related osteonecrosis of the jaw? An experimental study in rats. Oral Surg Oral Med Oral Pathol Oral Radiol 2014;117:329–34.

35. Del Fabbro M, Gallesio G, Mozzati M. Autologous platelet concentrates for bisphosphonate-related osteonecrosis of the jaw treatment and prevention. A systematic review of the literature. Eur J Cancer 2015;51(1):62–74.

36. Kuroshima S, Kovacic B, Kozloff K, et al. Intra-oral PTH administration promotes tooth extraction socket healing. J Dent Res 2013;92(6):553–9.

37. Hillstein J, Adler R, Edwards B, et al. Managing the care of patients receiving antiresorptive therapy for prevention and treatment of osteoporosis, executive summary of recommendations from the American Dental Association and Council on Scientific Affairs. J Am Dent Assoc 2011;142(11):1243–51.

38. Jadu F, Lee L, Pharoah M, et al. A retrospective study assessing the incidence, risk factors and co-morbidities of pamidronate-related necrosis of the jaws in multiple myeloma patients. Ann Oncol 2007;18(12):2015–9.

39. Marx RE, Sawatari Y, Fortin M, et al. Bisphosphonate-induced exposed bone (osteonecrosis/osteopetrosis)

of the jaws: risk factors, recognition, prevention, and treatment. J Oral Maxillofac Surg 2005;63(11):1567–75.

40. Saussez S, Javadian R, Hupin C, et al. Bisphosphonate-related osteonecrosis of the jaw and its associated risk factors: a Belgian case series. Laryngoscope 2009;119(2):323–9.

41. Tsao C, Darby I, Ebeling P, et al. Oral health risk factors for bisphosphonate-associated jaw osteonecrosis. J Oral Maxillofac Surg 2013;71:1360–6.

42. Khan A, Morrison A, Hanley D, et al. Diagnosis and management of osteonecrosis of the jaw: a systematic review and international consensus. J Bone Miner Res 2015;30(1):3–23.

43. McClung M, Harris S, Miller P, et al. Bisphosphonate therapy for osteoporosis: benefits, risks, and drug holiday. Am J Med 2013;126:13–20.

44. Damm D, Jones D. Bisphosphonate-related osteonecrosis of the jaws: a potential alternative to drug holidays. Gen Dent 2013;61(5):33–8.

Pharmacogenetics of Bisphosphonate-associated Osteonecrosis of the Jaw

P.L. Fung, BDS, MSc, PhD[a], P. Nicoletti, MD, PhD[b],
Y. Shen, MD, PhD[b,c], S. Porter, MD, PhD, FDS RCS, FDS RCSE[a],
S. Fedele, DDS, PhD[a,d,*]

KEYWORDS

- Jaw osteonecrosis • Bisphosphonates • Pharmacogenetics • Pharmacogenomics • Genes
- Single-nucleotide polymorphisms

KEY POINTS

- Osteonecrosis of the jaws (ONJ) develops in a small subgroup of individuals exposed to bisphosphonate medications.
- Although several associated clinical risk factors have been identified, it remains difficult to predict which individuals will develop ONJ.
- Pharmacogenetics has the potential to identify genetic variants associated with an increased risk (susceptibility) of developing ONJ.
- Several genome-wide association and candidate gene studies have been performed during the last few years; however, they are limited by small cohort size and lack of robust genomic statistical significance.
- The study of genetic susceptibility to ONJ requires international multicentre collaborative networks and larger and better phenotyped cohorts.

INTRODUCTION

Bisphosphonates (BPs) are antiresorptive agents commonly used in the treatment of osteoporosis, multiple myeloma, and bone metastases from solid cancers.[1] BPs are internalized into osteoclasts via endocytosis and result in the inhibition of osteoclast activity through different mechanisms.[2,3] Nitrogen-containing BPs, including alendronate, ibandronate, risedronate, pamidronate, and zoledronate, inhibit farnesyl pyrophosphate synthase, a key enzyme of the mevalonate pathway. This (1) prevents prenylation of guanosine triphosphatase (GTPase), which is essential for osteoclast function and survival, and (2) causes accumulation of isopentenyl diphosphate, which in turn can induce osteoclast apoptosis.[4] Non–nitrogen-containing BPs, including clodronate and etidronate,

Disclosure: The authors have nothing to disclose.
[a] UCL Eastman Dental Institute, University College London, 256 Gray's Inn Road, London WC1X 8LD, UK;
[b] Department of Systems Biology, Irving Cancer Research Center, Columbia University, 1130 St. Nicholas Avenue, New York, NY 10032, USA; [c] Department of Biomedical Informatics, Irving Cancer Research Center, Columbia University, 1130 St. Nicholas Avenue, New York, NY 10032, USA; [d] NIHR Biomedical Research Centre, University College London Hospitals, 149 Tottenham Court Road, London W1T 7DN, UK
* Corresponding author. Eastman Dental Institute and Hospital, University College London Hospitals Trust, University College London, 256 Gray's Inn Road, London WC1X 8LD, UK.
E-mail address: s.fedele@ucl.ac.uk

Oral Maxillofacial Surg Clin N Am 27 (2015) 537–546
http://dx.doi.org/10.1016/j.coms.2015.06.005
1042-3699/15/$ – see front matter © 2015 Elsevier Inc. All rights reserved.

are incorporated into an adenosine triphosphate analogue, which can also induce osteoclast apoptosis.[5]

BPs are associated with a potentially severe adverse drug reaction (ADR): osteonecrosis of the jaw (ONJ), which was initially reported in 2003.[6] Since then, thousands of ONJ cases have been reported worldwide.[7] ONJ is characterized by the development of jawbone necrosis and is traditionally presented with areas of exposed necrotic jawbone through mucosal or facial skin fenestrations ranging from a few millimeters to several centimeters.[8–10] More recent studies have reported that in approximately 25% of cases ONJ can also present without soft tissue fenestration (nonexposed variant), with affected patients showing otherwise unexplained painful symptoms, intraoral or extraoral fistulae, tooth mobility or tooth loss, sinusitis, or mandibular facture.[1,11–13] Both the exposed and nonexposed variants of ONJ can present with extensive necrosis, secondary infection, and severe pain,[14] therefore causing a significant reduction in the quality of life.[15] Figures on ONJ prevalence and incidence vary widely and remain controversial. Available data suggest that ONJ develops in a subgroup of individuals who use or have used BPs: approximately 7% among those using intravenous BPs for cancer management and 0.12% of those who take oral BPs because of osteoporosis.[16] Little robust information is available regarding ONJ etiopathogenesis; similarly, it is unclear why ONJ develops only in a subset of patients.[17,18] Several clinical risk factors have been associated with ONJ development, including underlying malignant disease, use of intravenous high-potency BPs, high-dose or long-term BP therapy, use of concomitant medications, dental infections, and surgical procedures to the jawbones.[19] Nevertheless, relevant literature lacks robustness and consistency, and in most instances ONJ remains an unpredictable ADR.

Interindividual genetic variants are known to potentially determine disparate response to medications, including toxicity. It was estimated that genetic variability could contribute to ADR development in more than half of the medications examined in a systematic review.[20] Interindividual genetic variability can therefore contribute to explaining ONJ development in a subset of individuals using BPs. In the past few years, several small studies have investigated the potential association of ONJ development with genetic factors.[21–31] This article provides a critical and comprehensive review of the available evidence regarding pharmacogenetics of ONJ.

PHARMACOGENETICS AND ADVERSE DRUG REACTIONS

Pharmacogenetics is the study of how genetic differences influence the variability in patients' responses to drugs, including toxicity.[32] Examples of genetic factors contributing to individuals' susceptibility to ADR include HLA-A*31:01 for carbamazepine (CMZ)-induced skin reactions in Europeans,[33] HLA-B*15:02 for CMZ-induced Stevens-Johnson syndrome in Asians,[34] SLCO1B1 for statin-induced myopathy,[35] and HLA-B*57:01 for abacavir-induced hypersensitivity reactions,[36,37] as well as for flucloxacillin-induced liver injury.[38] In most cases, the genetic risk variants are drug specific (1 or a few medications) and population (ethnicity) specific.[33,34,39] Among the drug-induced liver injuries, HLA-B*57:01 is only known to be associated with flucloxacillin-induced reactions, although HLA-DRB1*15:01 is known to be associated with both amoxicillin-clavulanate[39] and lumiracoxib.[40] Examples of successful and cost-effective translation of pharmacogenetic data into clinical practice include HLA-B*57:01 screening before initiating treatment with abacavir and HLA-B*15:02 screening before CMZ therapy in Asians, both recommended by the US Food and Drug Administration.[41,42] With such robust and growing evidence, pharmacogenetics is becoming a realistic mean to tailor and personalize safe and effective therapy for single individuals.[43] Pharmacogenetic studies comprise genome-wide association studies (GWASs) and candidate gene studies.[44] A total of 2 GWASs and 9 candidate gene studies have been performed in relation to ONJ.

GENOME-WIDE ASSOCIATION STUDIES ON OSTEONECROSIS OF THE JAW

GWAS is a comprehensive research approach that is useful for investigating both complex disease and drug response, including ADR. Typically, a GWAS screens millions of single-nucleotide polymorphisms (SNPs) across the entire genome, in which an SNP refers to a single-base difference in DNA sequence present in at least 1% of the general population.[45] The large set of SNPs, which form part of a standard GWAS genotyping chip, have been chosen based on their property of being proxies to others within the same genomic region; this is known as linkage disequilibrium (LD).[32] A successful GWAS relies on a reasonably complete coverage of genetic variants, which include SNPs that are typed with a chip, as well as SNPs that have not been typed but can be predicted through LD; a causal variant can be a typed SNP, or an untyped one with a typed proxy SNP. In the latter case, fine-mapping studies should follow to search for the untyped causal variant in the same genomic region. GWAS usually have case-control design and an SNP is identified as a risk factor if the frequency of its minor allele in the cases is significantly different than the controls. Because GWASs test millions of SNPs, it is possible that some variants are identified as having high frequency and very small P-values simply by chance; in order to avoid these false-positives, a stringent statistical correction for multiple comparisons is commonly required, which is known as Bonferroni correction. Instead of the usual $P<.05$, the significance level for GWAS is calculated as .05 divided by roughly 1 million SNPs (ie, $P<5E-08$).[45]

To date, 2 GWASs have been conducted on ONJ and relevant results are summarized in **Table 1**. The first GWAS, also the first pharmacogenetic study on ONJ, was published in 2008 by a Spanish team.[21] They studied 87 pamidronate-treated patients with multiple myeloma, who were of Spanish descent, of whom 22 had developed ONJ. These cases were compared with 65 drug-exposed controls who had not developed ONJ after a median follow-up of 64 months; 500,568 SNPs were screened and rs1934951 in *CYP2C8* was the most significant, although it did not reach genome-wide threshold of significance (odds ratio [OR], 12.75; 95% confidence interval [CI], 3.7–43.5; $P = 1.07E-06$). This study suggests that individuals with this SNP had nearly 13 times greater odds of developing ONJ than those without it. Although not directly affecting BP metabolism, *CYP2C8* is known to be involved in osteoclast inhibition, osteoblast differentiation, and regulation of vascular tone, which may contribute to ONJ development.[46]

The second GWAS was published in 2012 and compared 30 zoledronate-treated patients with breast cancer who had developed ONJ with 17 drug-exposed controls and 1726 population controls.[28] The participants were of European descent. Compared with the previous GWAS, 731,442 SNPs were screened. Standard imputation was performed to enrich the genotype data set, and an imputed SNP, rs17024608 in *RBMS3*, was found to be associated with ONJ, with borderline genome-wide significance (OR, 5.8; 95% CI, 3.0–11.0; $P = 7.47E-08$). The rs17024608 carriers had approximately 6 times higher odds of developing ONJ than the noncarriers. *RBMS3* is a gene involved in bone turnover and has been found to be associated with decreased bone mass and osteoporotic fracture.[28] *CYP2C8* variants were not confirmed as

risk factors for ONJ in this cohort of patients with breast cancer.

In summary, only 2 GWASs have been published so far and they suggest that variants in genes *CYP2C8* and *RBMS3*, which are both related to bone turnover, may be associated with ONJ development in patients of Spanish descent with multiple myeloma and in patients of European descent with breast cancer respectively. There are significant differences between these studies with regard to cohort size, case/control ratio, participants' ethnicity, underlying diseases, and BP type, which hinder meaningful comparison and data pooling. Also, both had a small number of cases, which limits their power to detect variants with high relative risk and represents the most likely cause for their failure to identify genome-wide significant variants. Another important aspect of GWASs is the need to replicate results in an independent population with similar phenotype, which is considered the gold standard approach so to minimizing the risk that potential technical or methodological bias could determine a spurious association signal.[47,48] A small number of candidate gene studies and 1 meta-analysis were designed to replicate association with rs1934951 in *CYP2C8* (discussed later), whereas there remains no attempted replication of rs17024608 in *RBMS3*.

CANDIDATE GENE STUDIES ON OSTEONECROSIS OF THE JAW

Similar to GWASs, candidate gene studies often have a case-control design.[49] In general they focus on potentially biologically relevant genes; for ADR, most of the established and high-risk genetic risk factors are relevant to drug metabolism or transporters genes.[39] In contrast with GWASs, candidate gene studies screen much fewer variants and do not represent a hypothesis-free approach.[50] They are also prone to methodological weaknesses because they typically have small cohort size, no Bonferroni correction for the P-value, and often do not correct for the ethnicity of the cohort. Therefore, it has been suggested that candidate gene design is more suitable for replication studies.[51] A total of 9 candidate gene studies on ONJ were published between 2010 and 2013,[22–27,29–31] including both replication and discovery gene studies.

Replication Candidate Gene Studies

Four candidate gene studies attempted to replicate the results of the Spanish GWAS[21] through investigating the possible association between rs1934951 in *CYP2C8* and ONJ in their respective independent cohorts (**Table 2**).[22,23,27,30] All studies

Table 1
Summary of GWAS

Year	Population	Underlying Disease	BP Type	Cases (n)	Controls (n)	Genotyping	SNP	Gene	Chr	P-Value	OR (95% CI)	Ref
2008	Spanish	Multiple myeloma	Most on pamidronate Zoledronate	22	65 BPs controls	Affymetrix GeneChip Mapping 500K set 500,568 SNPs screened	rs1934951	CYP2C8	10	1.07E-06	12.75 (3.7–43.5)	21
							rs1934980	CYP2C8	10	4.23E-06	13.88 (4.0–46.7)	
							rs1341162	CYP2C8	10	6.22E-06	13.27 (3.5–49.9)	
							rs17110453	CYP2C8	10	2.15E-05	10.2 (3.2–32.1)	
2012	North-western, southern, eastern European descent	Osteoporosis Breast cancer	Most on zoledronate	30	17 BPs controls 1726 population controls	Illumina Human Omni Express 12v1.0 chip 731,442 SNPs analyzed	rs17024608	RBMS3	3	7.47E-08	5.8 (3.0–11.0)	28
							rs5768434	FAM19A5	22	1.17E-07	12.6 (4.9–32.2)	
							rs11064477	PHB2	12	5.16E-07	21.7 (6.5–71.9)	
							12–7016684	C1S	12	5.85E-07	21.1 (6.4–69.8)	
							8–58133986	IMPAD1	8	3.10E-06	7.3 (3.1–16.9)	
							rs1886629	KCNT2	1	5.53E-06	3.6 (2.1–6.5)	
							rs7588295	CSRNP3	2	6.24E-06	8.6 (3.3–22.17)	
							rs4431170	MARCH1	4	7.28E-06	5.1 (2.5–10.6)	
							rs7740004	C6orf170	6	7.87E-06	5.9 (2.7–13.0)	
							rs11189381	SFRP5	10	8.17E-06	6.8 (2.9–15.8)	
							rs12903202	ALDH1A2	15	9.15E-06	4.0 (2.1–7.4)	
							rs17751934	MEX3C	18	9.16E-06	5.0 (2.4–10.1)	
							11–23990403	LUZP2	11	9.94E-06	12.7 (4.0–36.8)	

Abbreviations: Chr, chromosome; CI, confidence interval; OR, odds ratio.

Data from Sarasquete ME, García-Sanz R, Marín L, et al. Bisphosphonate-related osteonecrosis of the jaw is associated with polymorphisms of the cytochrome P450 CYP2C8 in multiple myeloma: a genome-wide single nucleotide polymorphism analysis. Blood 2008;112(7):2709–12; and Nicoletti P, Cartsos VM, Palaska PK, et al. Genomewide pharmacogenetics of bisphosphonate-induced osteonecrosis of the jaw: the role of RBMS3. Oncologist 2012;17(2):279–87.

Table 2
Summary of candidate gene replication studies on CYP2C8

Year	Population	Underlying Disease	BP Type	Cases (n)	Controls (n)	Genotyping	SNP	Gene	Chr	P-Value	OR (95% CI)	Ref
2010	80% White 10% African American	Prostate cancer	Zoledronate Combination of BPs	17	83 BPs controls	Big Dye Terminator Cycle Sequencing Ready Reaction kit V3.1	rs1934951	CYP2C8	10	>.47	0.63 (0.17–2.42)	22
2011	68% White 24% African American	Multiple myeloma	Zoledronate and/or pamidronate	12	66 BPs controls	Taqman Pyrosequencing	rs1934951 rs1934980	CYP2C8 CYP2C8	10 10	.63 .66	0.68 (0.14–3.22) 0.70 (0.15–3.36)	23
2011	White	Multiple myeloma	Zoledronate	42	37 BPs controls 45 population controls	Taqman	rs1934951	CYP2C8	10	.13	—	27
2012	Hungarian	Breast cancer Osteoporosis Multiple myeloma Prostate cancer	Zoledronate Ibandronate Pamidronate	46	224 population controls	Taqman	rs1934951	CYP2C8	10	>.05		30

Data from Refs.[22,23,27,30]

failed to confirm that this variant is significantly associated with the trait (P>.05). Paradoxically, Katz and colleagues[23] and English and colleagues[22] reported a protective OR for this variant. These apparently contradicting results are likely to be related to the design of the replication studies, which failed to investigate populations phenotypically and ethnically similar to that of the original discovery study. In contrast with the first GWAS, none of the 4 studies included individuals of Spanish descent, although their cohorts consisted mainly of white caucasian participants; African Americans were also inappropriately included.[22,23] Also, all 4 cohorts were predominantly exposed to zoledronate instead of pamidronate. Further, only 2 replication studies focused on patients with multiple myeloma,[23,27] whereas 1 recruited individuals with metastatic prostate cancer,[22] and 1 included individuals with osteoporosis and a wide range of malignant disorders.[30] A recent meta-analysis by Zhong and colleagues[52] attempted data pooling from the 4 candidate gene replication studies and the discovery Spanish GWAS. They confirmed that rs1934951 in CYP2C8 is not associated with ONJ across the whole merged population (OR, 2.05; 95% CI, 0.67–6.29; P = .2), but it might be associated with ONJ development in patients with multiple myeloma with a dominant effect (OR, 5.77; 95% CI, 1.21–27.63; P = .03; combined effect from only 2 studies[21,27]). Better-designed studies are required for appropriate replication of rs1934951. There remains no published attempted replication of rs17024608.

Discovery Candidate Gene Studies

Six discovery candidate gene studies investigated variants in genes other than CYP2C8 and are summarized in **Table 3**.[23–26,29,31] These studies analyzed the separate and combined effects of variants located in several genes, which had been chosen because they may relate to BP metabolism and/or ONJ pathogenesis (eg, bone turnover). Most of them screened only a small number of variants and had small cohorts, and are therefore susceptible to methodological limitations such as inadequate power. None of the SNPs tested reached the genome-wide significance level (ie, P<5E-08).

The largest discovery candidate gene study in the literature compared 94 ONJ cases with 110 ethnicity-matched BP-exposed controls.[31] The cohort included individuals with malignant disorders, including multiple myeloma, breast cancer, and prostate cancer, who had been exposed mainly to zoledronate or pamidronate. The study

hypothesis was that ONJ susceptibility might be linked to the major histocompatibility complex (MHC) class II system, which encodes HLA class II alleles. As mentioned earlier, HLA alleles are major genetic risk factors for ADRs and are also associated with the adaptive immune system and infection, which in the case of ONJ may be related to the antigen-presenting function of osteoclasts and increased infection and/or inflammation.[17] According to the significance threshold set by the study, 2 independent HLA haplotypes, DRB1*01/DRB1*15 and DQB1*05:01/DQB1*06:02, were significantly associated with ONJ development (uncorrected P≤.05), with OR greater than 2. Moreover, the association seemed to be stronger when more than 1 haplotype was considered together (OR, 3; corrected P = .0003).[31] An Italian study by Arduino and colleagues[24] recruited a population of 30 women with breast cancer or multiple myeloma who had developed zoledronate-induced ONJ; 30 controls without ONJ matched for drug, gender, disease, and ethnicity, as well as 125 healthy controls. The candidate gene of this study was vascular endothelial growth factor (VEGF), which had previously been reported to be associated with avascular osteonecrosis of the femoral head.[53,54] No statistically significant association was found for any of the 3 studied SNPs (−634 G>C, +936 C>T, and −2578 C>A; P>.05). However, the haplotype determined by rs2010963 and rs699947 was significantly associated with ONJ (corrected P = .02). Another Italian study by La Ferla and colleagues[29] studied 30 zoledronate-induced ONJ cases and 53 zoledronate-exposed controls with multiple myeloma, breast cancer, and prostate cancer. Participants were tested for 3 candidate polymorphisms, including 1 aromatase and 2 estrogen receptor polymorphisms, which were selected because of their reported effects on bone mineral density and remodeling. Results showed that rs10046 (g.132810 C > T), a polymorphism in gene CYP19A1, was more prevalent among ONJ cases (OR, 2.83; P = .04). Marini and colleagues[26] recruited 64 Italian patients with multiple myeloma, breast cancer, and prostate cancer who had received zoledronate, 34 of whom developed ONJ. They studied polymorphism rs2297480 in gene FDPS (farnesyl pyrophosphate synthase, a key enzyme of the mevalonate pathway of osteoclasts), which was significantly associated with ONJ (P = .03), although it did not have genome-wide significance. This study represents the first attempt to investigate a candidate gene directly involved in BPs' mechanism of action. Katz and colleagues[23] recruited patients with multiple myeloma only, including 12 ONJ cases and 66

Table 3
Summary of discovery candidate gene studies

Year	Population	Underlying Disease	BPs Type	Case (n)	Control (n)	Genotyping	SNP	Gene	Chr	P-Value	OR (95% CI)	Ref
2011	68% White 24% African American	MM	ZOL and/or PM	12	66 BPs controls	Taqman Pyrosequencing	rs1800012	COL1A1	17	.55	1.69 (0.30–9.70)	23
							rs12458117	RANK	18	.38	2.14 (0.39–11.71)	
							rs243865	MMP2	16	.11	3.49 (0.75–16.18)	
							rs2073618	OPG	8	.38	2.16 (0.38–12.23)	
							rs3102735	OPG	8	.75	0.79 (0.19–3.34)	
							rs11730582	OPN	4	.21	2.97 (0.53–16.55)	
							rs28357094	OPN	4	.41	0.51 (0.10–2.59)	
							rs1800629	TNF	6	.67	0.68 (0.12–3.95)	
2011	Italian	BC, MM	ZOL	30	30 BPs controls 125 population controls	Taqman	rs3025039	VEGF	6	.40	0.57 (0.21–1.54)	24
							rs699947			.78	0.99 (0.31–3.18)	
							rs2010963			.86	0.96 (0.37–2.53)	
2011	NA	MM	ZOL	9	10 BPs controls	Affymetrix DMET plus platform 1936 SNPs analyzed	rs1152003	PPARG	3	.0055	—	25
							rs10893	ABP1	7	.023		
							rs4725373			.023		
							rs1049793			.023		
							rs2463437	CHST11	12	.0198		
							rs903247			.0198		
							rs2468110			.0198		
							rs2097937	CROT	7	.0198		
2011	White	BC, MM, PC	ZOL	34	34 BPs controls	GoTaq	rs2297480	FDPS	1	.03	—	26
2012	White	BC, MM, PC	ZOL	30	53 BPs controls	Taqman	rs2234693	ESR1	6	>.05	—	29
							rs9340799	ESR1	6	>.05	—	
							rs10046	CYP19A1	15	.0439	2.83	
2013	White	BC, MM, PC	ZOL or PM or combination of BPs	94	110 BPs controls	LABType single strand oligonucleotide typing kit	DRB1*01	MHC	6	.049	2.0 (0.99–4.1)	31
							DRB1*15			.014	2.3 (1.2–4.4)	
							DQB1*05:01			.050	2.0 (0.99–4.0)	
							DQB1*06:02			.014	2.3 (1.2–4.6)	

Abbreviations: BC, breast cancer; DMET, drug metabolism enzymes and transporters; MM, multiple myeloma; NA, not available; PC, prostate cancer; PM, pamidronate; ZOL, zoledronate.
Data from Refs.[23–26,29,31]

controls, who were managed with zoledronate and/or pamidronate. In addition to gene *CYP2C8*, 6 other candidate genes were studied based on their potential roles in osteoclast genesis and differentiation, bone resorption, and bone mineral density. The results showed that, per se, all candidate genes had no effects on ONJ, although a combined genotype of *COL1A1*, *RANK*, *MMP2*, *OPG*, and *OPN* was significantly associated with ONJ development (OR, 1.2; 95% CI, 1.8–69.9; *P* = .0097).

Di Martino and colleagues[25] studied 1936 SNPs relevant to 225 genes associated with drug metabolism, disposition, and transport in 9 patients with multiple myeloma and ONJ treated with zoledronate and 10 matched controls. The investigators claimed that using a platform that interrogates only highly selective SNPs has the advantage of avoiding an extremely high number of comparisons, and therefore avoids the need for statistical corrections and large patient cohorts. As a consequence, the study adopted an uncorrected significance level of *P*<.05 and reported that variants in 4 genes, *PPARG*, *ABP1*, *CHST11*, and *CROT*, were statistically significant. However, because nearly 2000 SNPs were screened, Bonferroni correction was required and the significance threshold should be approximately 2.5E-5 instead (ie, 0.05 divided by 1936),[55] which would mean that no SNPs reached the corrected significance threshold. Nonetheless, from uncorrected results, patients with rs1152003, the top SNP in *PPARG*, had more than 30 times higher odds of developing ONJ (OR, 31.5; 95% CI, 2.35–422.32; *P* = .0055). *PPARG* has also been associated with bone remodeling, bone mass density, as well as angiogenesis.[25]

In summary, because of small sample sizes and other methodological limitations, there remains little robust evidence that ONJ development is associated with any of the candidate SNPs or genes considered in available studies.

SUMMARY

There are several available pharmacogenetic studies on ONJ, which are characterized by small sample sizes and mainly represent candidate gene analyses. Although GWASs are considered more powerful than candidate gene studies because of wider genome coverage and the advantage of being hypothesis free, there are currently only 2 GWASs on ONJ phenotype, which only investigated a modest number of cases and have not been appropriately replicated. Overall, no genome-wide significant variant has been robustly associated with the susceptibility to ONJ. In addition to the methodological limitations mentioned earlier, this may suggests that, if there is any genetic predisposition, it may be caused by common variants with moderate effect size, or rare variants. In the search for genome-wide significant SNPs for ONJ, international multicentre collaborative networks are required in order to study larger and better phenotyped cohorts.

REFERENCES

1. Ruggiero SL, Dodson TB, Fantasia J, et al, American Association of Oral and Maxillofacial Surgeons. American Association of Oral and Maxillofacial Surgeons position paper on medication-related osteonecrosis of the jaw–2014 update. J Oral Maxillofac Surg 2014;72(10):1938–56.
2. Cremers S, Papapoulos S. Pharmacology of bisphosphonates. Bone 2011;49(1):42–9.
3. Russell RG. Bisphosphonates: mode of action and pharmacology. Pediatrics 2007;119(Suppl 2): S150–62.
4. Russell RG. Bisphosphonates: the first 40years. Bone 2011;49(1):2–19.
5. Rogers MJ, Crockett JC, Coxon FP, et al. Biochemical and molecular mechanisms of action of bisphosphonates. Bone 2011;49(1):34–41.
6. Marx RE. Pamidronate (Aredia) and zoledronate (Zometa) induced avascular necrosis of the jaws: a growing epidemic. J Oral Maxillofac Surg 2003; 61(9):1115–7.
7. Filleul O, Crompot E, Saussez S. Bisphosphonate-induced osteonecrosis of the jaw: a review of 2,400 patient cases. J Cancer Res Clin Oncol 2010;136(8):1117–24.
8. Sambrook P, Olver I, Goss A. Bisphosphonates and osteonecrosis of the jaw. Aust Fam Physician 2006; 35(10):801–3.
9. Khosla S, Burr D, Cauley J, et al. Bisphosphonate-associated osteonecrosis of the jaw: report of a task force of the American Society for Bone and Mineral Research. J Bone Miner Res 2007;22(10): 1479–91.
10. Ruggiero SL, Dodson TB, Assael LA, et al. American Association of Oral and Maxillofacial Surgeons position paper on bisphosphonate-related osteonecrosis of the jaws–2009 update. J Oral Maxillofac Surg 2009;67(5 Suppl):2–12.
11. Fedele S, Porter SR, D'Aiuto F, et al. Nonexposed variant of bisphosphonate-associated osteonecrosis of the jaw: a case series. Am J Med 2010;123(11): 1060–4.
12. Bedogni A, Fusco V, Agrillo A, et al. Learning from experience. Proposal of a refined definition and staging system for bisphosphonate-related osteonecrosis of the jaw (BRONJ). Oral Dis 2012;18(6): 621–3.

13. Fedele S, Bedogni G, Scoletta M, et al. Up to a quarter of patients with osteonecrosis of the jaw associated with antiresorptive agents remain undiagnosed. Br J Oral Maxillofac Surg 2015; 53(1):13–7.

14. Bagan JV, Hens-Aumente E, Leopoldo-Rodado M, et al. Bisphosphonate-related osteonecrosis of the jaws: study of the staging system in a series of clinical cases. Oral Oncol 2012;48(8):753–7.

15. Miksad RA, Lai KC, Dodson TB, et al. Quality of life implications of bisphosphonate-associated osteonecrosis of the jaw. Oncologist 2011;16(1):121–32.

16. Kühl S, Walter C, Acham S, et al. Bisphosphonate-related osteonecrosis of the jaws–a review. Oral Oncol 2012;48(10):938–47.

17. Landesberg R, Woo V, Cremers S, et al. Potential pathophysiological mechanisms in osteonecrosis of the jaw. Ann N Y Acad Sci 2011;1218:62–79.

18. Allen MR. The effects of bisphosphonates on jaw bone remodeling, tissue properties, and extraction healing. Odontology 2011;99(1):8–17.

19. Khan AA, Sándor GK, Dore E, et al. Bisphosphonate associated osteonecrosis of the jaw. J Rheumatol 2009;36(3):478–90.

20. Phillips KA, Veenstra DL, Oren E, et al. Potential role of pharmacogenomics in reducing adverse drug reactions: a systematic review. JAMA 2001; 286(18):2270–9.

21. Sarasquete ME, García-Sanz R, Marín L, et al. Bisphosphonate-related osteonecrosis of the jaw is associated with polymorphisms of the cytochrome P450 CYP2C8 in multiple myeloma: a genomewide single nucleotide polymorphism analysis. Blood 2008;112(7):2709–12.

22. English BC, Baum CE, Adelberg DE, et al. A SNP in CYP2C8 is not associated with the development of bisphosphonate-related osteonecrosis of the jaw in men with castrate-resistant prostate cancer. Ther Clin Risk Manag 2010;6:579–83.

23. Katz J, Gong Y, Salmasinia D, et al. Genetic polymorphisms and other risk factors associated with bisphosphonate induced osteonecrosis of the jaw. Int J Oral Maxillofac Surg 2011;40(6):605–11.

24. Arduino PG, Menegatti E, Scoletta M, et al. Vascular endothelial growth factor genetic polymorphisms and haplotypes in female patients with bisphosphonate-related osteonecrosis of the jaws. J Oral Pathol Med 2011;40(6):510–5.

25. Di Martino MT, Arbitrio M, Guzzi PH, et al. A peroxisome proliferator-activated receptor gamma (PPARG) polymorphism is associated with zoledronic acid-related osteonecrosis of the jaw in multiple myeloma patients: analysis by DMET microarray profiling. Br J Haematol 2011;154(4):529–33.

26. Marini F, Tonelli P, Cavalli L, et al. Pharmacogenetics of bisphosphonate-associated osteonecrosis of the jaw. Front Biosci (Elite Ed) 2011;3:364–70.

27. Such E, Cervera J, Terpos E, et al. CYP2C8 gene polymorphism and bisphosphonate-related osteonecrosis of the jaw in patients with multiple myeloma. Haematologica 2011;96(10):1557–9.

28. Nicoletti P, Cartsos VM, Palaska PK, et al. Genomewide pharmacogenetics of bisphosphonate-induced osteonecrosis of the jaw: the role of RBMS3. Oncologist 2012;17(2):279–87.

29. La Ferla F, Paolicchi E, Crea F, et al. An aromatase polymorphism (g.132810C>T) predicts risk of bisphosphonate-related osteonecrosis of the jaw. Biomark Med 2012;6(2):201–9.

30. Balla B, Vaszilko M, Kósa JP, et al. New approach to analyze genetic and clinical data in bisphosphonate-induced osteonecrosis of the jaw. Oral Dis 2012;18(6):580–5.

31. Stockmann P, Nkenke E, Englbrecht M, et al. Major histocompatibility complex class II polymorphisms are associated with the development of antiresorptive agent-induced osteonecrosis of the jaw. J Craniomaxillofac Surg 2013;41(1):71–5.

32. Roses AD. Pharmacogenetics and the practice of medicine. Nature 2000;405(6788):857–65.

33. McCormack M, Alfirevic A, Bourgeois S, et al. HLA-A*3101 and carbamazepine-induced hypersensitivity reactions in Europeans. N Engl J Med 2011; 364(12):1134–43.

34. Chung WH, Hung SI, Hong HS, et al. Medical genetics: a marker for Stevens-Johnson syndrome. Nature 2004;428(6982):486.

35. Link E, Parish S, Armitage J, et al. SLCO1B1 variants and statin-induced myopathy–a genomewide study. N Engl J Med 2008;359(8):789–99.

36. Mallal S, Nolan D, Witt C, et al. Association between presence of HLA-B*5701, HLA-DR7, and HLA-DQ3 and hypersensitivity to HIV-1 reverse-transcriptase inhibitor abacavir. Lancet 2002;359(9308):727–32.

37. Hetherington S, Hughes AR, Mosteller M, et al. Genetic variations in HLA-B region and hypersensitivity reactions to abacavir. Lancet 2002;359(9312): 1121–2.

38. Daly AK, Donaldson PT, Bhatnagar P, et al. HLA-B*5701 genotype is a major determinant of drug-induced liver injury due to flucloxacillin. Nat Genet 2009;41(7):816–9.

39. Daly AK. Pharmacogenomics of adverse drug reactions. Genome Med 2013;5(1):5.

40. Singer JB, Lewitzky S, Leroy E, et al. A genomewide study identifies HLA alleles associated with lumiracoxib-related liver injury. Nat Genet 2010; 42(8):711–4.

41. Mallal S, Phillips E, Carosi G, et al, PREDICT-1 Study Team. HLA-B*5701 screening for hypersensitivity to abacavir. N Engl J Med 2008;358(6):568–79.

42. Leckband SG, Kelsoe JR, Dunnenberger HM, et al, Clinical Pharmacogenetics Implementation Consortium. Clinical Pharmacogenetics Implementation

Consortium guidelines for HLA-B genotype and carbamazepine dosing. Clin Pharmacol Ther 2013; 94(3):324–8.

43. Hamburg MA, Collins FS. The path to personalized medicine. N Engl J Med 2010;363(4):301–4.

44. Daly AK. Genome-wide association studies in pharmacogenomics. Nat Rev Genet 2010;11(4):241–6.

45. Daly AK. Using genome-wide association studies to identify genes important in serious adverse drug reactions. Annu Rev Pharmacol Toxicol 2012;52:21–35.

46. Sarasquete ME, González M, San Miguel JF, et al. Bisphosphonate-related osteonecrosis: genetic and acquired risk factors. Oral Dis 2009;15(6):382–7.

47. Bush WS, Moore JH. Chapter 11: genome-wide association studies. PLoS Comput Biol 2012;8(12): e1002822.

48. McCarthy MI, Abecasis GR, Cardon LR, et al. Genome-wide association studies for complex traits: consensus, uncertainty and challenges. Nat Rev Genet 2008;9(5):356–69.

49. Daly AK, Day CP. Candidate gene case-control association studies: advantages and potential pitfalls. Br J Clin Pharmacol 2001;52(5):489–99.

50. Tabor HK, Risch NJ, Myers RM. Candidate-gene approaches for studying complex genetic traits: practical considerations. Nat Rev Genet 2002;3(5): 391–7.

51. Kraft P, Zeggini E, Ioannidis JP. Replication in genome-wide association studies. Stat Sci 2009; 24(4):561–73.

52. Zhong DN, Wu JZ, Li GJ. Association between CYP2C8 (rs1934951) polymorphism and bisphosphonate-related osteonecrosis of the jaws in patients on bisphosphonate therapy: a meta-analysis. Acta Haematol 2013;129(2):90–5.

53. Kim TH, Hong JM, Lee JY, et al. Promoter polymorphisms of the vascular endothelial growth factor gene is associated with an osteonecrosis of the femoral head in the Korean population. Osteoarthritis Cartilage 2008;16(3):287–91.

54. Lee YJ, Lee JS, Kang EH, et al. Vascular endothelial growth factor polymorphisms in patients with steroid-induced femoral head osteonecrosis. J Orthop Res 2012;30(1):21–7.

55. Rice TK, Schork NJ, Rao DC. Methods for handling multiple testing. Adv Genet 2008;60:293–308.

The Role of Antiangiogenic Therapy in the Development of Osteonecrosis of the Jaw

John E. Fantasia, DDS

KEYWORDS

- Antiangiogenic therapy • Vascular endothelial growth factor inhibitors • Tyrosine kinase inhibitors
- Mammalian target of rapamycin inhibitors • Nitrogen-containing bisphosphonates
- Receptor activator of nuclear factor-κB ligand inhibitors • Denosumab

KEY POINTS

- Osteonecrosis of the jaw (ONJ) has been linked to the use of various nitrogen-containing bisphosphonates and denosumab.
- Drugs that suppress angiogenesis also play a role in ONJ.
- Patients receiving antiresorptive medications and a medication with antiangiogenic properties are likely at increased risk for ONJ.
- Drugs with antiangiogenic properties include a monoclonal inhibitor of angiogenesis, and certain tyrosine kinase inhibitors, mammalian target of rapamycin inhibitors, and immunomodulatory agents.

INTRODUCTION

Medication-related osteonecrosis of the jaws (MRONJ) has primarily been associated with antiresorptive medications, specifically nitrogen-containing bisphosphonates (nBP) and the monoclonal inhibitor of the receptor activator of nuclear factor-κB ligand (denosumab). The pathogenesis of osteonecrosis of the jaw (ONJ) is likely multifactorial although impaired bone resorption certainly plays a crucial role, and the vasculature may also play a key role in the pathophysiology.[1] For review, the nBPs include alendronate (Fosamax), risedronate (Actonel, Atelvia), ibandronate (Boniva), pamidronate (Aredia), and zoledronic acid (ZA) (Zometa, Reclast). Denosumab is marketed as Prolia, for osteoporosis; and Xgeva, for prevention of skeletal-related events in patients with bone metastasis from solid tumors. The standard dosing of denosumab (Prolia) for osteoporosis is 60 mg subcutaneous injection every 6 months. The standard dosing of denosumab (Xgeva) for bone metastasis from solid tumors is 120 mg subcutaneous injection every 4 weeks. Recent studies have noted that angiogenesis suppression may play a role in developing ONJ and that serum vascular endothelial growth factor (VEGF) levels may be a predictive marker of ONJ.[2] Both nBPs and denosumab block bone destruction because they inhibit osteoclast-mediated bone resorption. nBPs are also known to inhibit angiogenesis.[3] To date, denosumab has not demonstrated antiangiogenic activity.[4] The development of MRONJ associated with bisphosphonates and denosumab exposure has been well documented.[5–7] In patients with certain cancers, nBP or denosumab is frequently used in

Division of Oral and Maxillofacial Pathology, Department of Dental Medicine, Hofstra North Shore-LIJ School of Medicine, 270-05 76th Avenue, New Hyde Park, NY 11040, USA
E-mail address: fantasia@lij.edu

Oral Maxillofacial Surg Clin N Am 27 (2015) 547–553
http://dx.doi.org/10.1016/j.coms.2015.06.004
1042-3699/15/$ – see front matter © 2015 Elsevier Inc. All rights reserved.

combination with medications that have antiangiogenic properties. Many traditional chemotherapeutic agents have antiangiogenic properties.[8] Data are emerging to show that either nBPs or denosumab in combination with targeted antiangiogenic therapies increases the likelihood of MRONJ.[9]

The past decade has seen increasing use of molecular targeted therapies for cancer and other disease processes. Angiogenesis is a rational target for therapy, as tumor growth and metastasis depends on neovascularization. These medications include use of the VEGF-specific antibody (bevacizumab) in combination with chemotherapy. Moreover, tyrosine kinase inhibitors (TKIs) that block the VEGF receptor and other kinases in both endothelial cells and cancer cells have yielded survival benefit in patients with some forms of cancer.[10] Examples of TKIs include sunitinib (Sutent) and sorafenib (Nexavar). There are isolated case reports and cohort studies suggesting an increased risk of ONJ occurring in patients treated with medications used in the treatment of various cancers and conditions that are antiangiogenic or targets of the VEGF pathway. Other classes of cancer drugs can have antiangiogenic properties. The mammalian target of rapamycin (mTOR) inhibitor everolimus has antiangiogenic properties distinct from a VEGF-receptor TKI.[11] Immunomodulatory agents such as thalidomide, which has been used in the treatment of multiple myeloma, also have antiangiogenic properties.[12] Most patients with cancer receive a variety of antineoplastic medications, and cancers with primary skeletal involvement, such as multiple myeloma, and other cancers with skeletal metastasis are treated with antiresorptive medications. This treatment complicates identification of the causative agent or agents responsible for osteonecrosis. There are evolving data to suggest an increased incidence of MRONJ and worsening of the condition in patients who are receiving an antiresorptive and a medication that also influences angiogenesis.[13] Prospective data are needed to help define whether the incidence of osteonecrosis is the same, additive, or synergistic when antiresorptive agents are used in combination with medications with antiangiogenic properties (**Table 1**).

MEDICATION-RELATED OSTEONECROSIS OF THE JAWS IN PATIENTS RECEIVING THE VASCULAR ENDOTHELIAL GROWTH FACTOR INHIBITOR BEVACIZUMAB, WITH AND WITHOUT ANTIRESORPTIVE EXPOSURE

Bevacizumab binds VEGF, and prevents the interaction of VEGF to its receptors on the surface of

Table 1
Medications, generic and proprietary names, used in the treatment of various cancers and conditions that are antiangiogenic or targets of the vascular endothelial growth factor pathway

Generic	Brand Name in USA	Form	Indications for Use
Monoclonal Antibody Inhibitor of Angiogenesis			
Bevacizumab	Avastin	IV infusion	mCRC, NSCLC, Glio, mRCC
Tyrosine Kinase Inhibitors (TKIs)			
Sunitinib	Sutent	Capsule	GIST, RCC, pNET
Sorafenib	Nexavar	Tablet	HCC, RCC
Panzopanib	Votrient	Tablet	RCC, STS
Axitinib	Inlyta	Tablet	RCC
Mammalian Target of Rapamycin (mTOR) Pathway Inhibitors			
Everolimus	Afinitor	Tablet	HR+BC, pNET, RCC, TSC, SEGA
Temsirolimus	Toriseliv	Infusion	RCC
Sirolimus	Rapamune	Tablet	Organ rejection in renal transplant
Immunomodulatory Agents			
Thalidomide	Thalomid	Capsule	MM, ENL
Lenalidomide	Revlimid	Capsule	MM, MDS, MCL
Pomalidomide	Pomalyst	Capsule	MM

Abbreviations: ENL, erythema nodosum leprosum; GIST, gastrointestinal stromal tumor; Glio, glioblastoma; HCC, hepatocellular carcinoma; HR+BC, hormone receptor–positive breast carcinoma; IV, intravenous; MCL, mantle cell lymphoma; mCRC, metastatic colorectal carcinoma; MDS, myelodysplastic syndrome; MM, multiple myeloma; mRCC, metastatic renal cell carcinoma; NSCLC, nonsquamous non–small cell lung carcinoma; pNET, pancreatic neuroendocrine tumor; RCC, renal cell carcinoma; SEGA, subependymal giant cell astrocytoma; STS, soft tissue sarcoma; TSC, tuberous sclerosis complex.

endothelial cells. The interaction of VEGF with its receptors leads to proliferation of endothelial cells and formation of new blood vessels. Bevacizumab causes reduction of microvascular growth and inhibition of metastatic disease progression. The primary indication for use has been with metastatic colorectal carcinoma, nonsquamous non–small cell lung cancer, glioblastoma, metastatic renal cell carcinoma (RCC), and persistent, recurrent, or metastatic carcinoma of the cervix.[14] The drug has also been used as an intravitreal injection in the treatment of macular degeneration.

In 2008, Estilo and colleagues[15] reported 2 cases of ONJ, the first of which was a 51-year-old woman with breast carcinoma had received 8 doses of bevacizumab, and 6 weeks after her last dose of bevacizumab she complained of lower jaw discomfort and bone protruding from the lower jaw. The second patient was a 33-year-old woman with glioblastoma multiforme treated with combination surgery/radiation therapy that did not include the oral cavity or jaw, and chemotherapy. She was placed on bevacizumab for 2 weeks, and 13 weeks later exposed mandibular bone consistent with ONJ was identified.[15] Greuter and colleagues[16] reported a 63-year-old woman with breast cancer treated with chemotherapy that included bevacizumab. One month after therapy she developed left maxillary pain resulting in extraction of the 2 left maxillary molars, and subsequent development of ONJ. Ayllon and colleagues[17] reported a female patient with breast cancer who received zoledronate and bevacizumab before developing ONJ. In 2009, Serra and colleagues[18] reported ONJ in a patient with lung adenocarcinoma who developed the condition after a dental extraction; bevacizumab was started 1 week after the extraction. In 2009, Christodoulou and colleagues[13] studied a cohort receiving bisphosphonates for osseous metastases with and without antiangiogenic therapy. Three patients developed ONJ: 2 patients with breast cancer and 1 with colorectal cancer who received the bisphosphonate, ibandronic acid or ZA, and bevacizumab. This study concluded that the combination of bisphosphonates and antiangiogenic factors induces ONJ more frequently than bisphosphonates alone. Guarneri and colleagues,[19] in a review of 3 large prospective trials in advanced breast cancer, identified 2 patients receiving bevacizumab who developed ONJ without exposure to bisphosphonates. The overall incidence of ONJ with bevacizumab therapy was 0.3% in the double-blinded phase of the 2 randomized trials and 0.4% in the single-arm study. These studies included patients exposed to bevacizumab alone and bevacizumab with bisphosphonate exposure. None of the patients in the pooled placebo arm

(no bevacizumab) experienced ONJ.[19] The data indicated that the overall incidence of ONJ in those receiving both bevacizumab and bisphosphonates were in the range of reported incidence of ONJ occurring in patients receiving bisphosphonates alone. Francini and colleagues[20] evaluated data on 59 patients, 34 with breast cancer and 25 with non–small cell lung cancer, who received ZA and bevacizumab. After a median follow-up of 19.7 months, none of the study participants developed ONJ.[20] A 2011 study by Ngamphaiboon and colleagues[21] reported on ONJ in patients with metastatic breast cancer treated with and without bevacizumab. The investigators identified 27 ONJ patients; 7 patients received bevacizumab and bisphosphonates and 20 patients received bisphosphonates alone. The focus of the study was to assess dental outcomes in the 2 groups. Hopp and colleagues[22] reported a 58-year-old man with retinal vascular thrombosis treated with intravitreal administration of bevacizumab who developed ONJ of the left lingual mandible. There was no history of bisphosphonate or long-term steroid therapy.[22] In 2012, Disel and colleagues[23] reported a case of ONJ in a patient with metastatic carcinoma of the sigmoid colon, with no history of bisphosphonate use, who received palliative chemotherapy that included bevacizumab. Bone exposure in the right posterior mandible occurred, and ONJ was confirmed with biopsy. Brunamonti Binello and colleagues[24] reported a case of ONJ of the left posterior mandible occurring in a patient with adenocarcinoma of the left parotid gland and bone metastasis treated with chemotherapy that included bevacizumab; there was no history of bisphosphonate exposure or radiation therapy treatments. Katsenos and colleagues[25] reported a 57-year-old man with non–small cell lung cancer presenting with bone metastasis. Treatment consisted of chemotherapy including bevacizumab and ZA, and ONJ developed 12 weeks after initiation of bevacizumab administration. These investigators attributed the cause of ONJ to bevacizumab, but commented that a possible synergic effect of the bisphosphonate could not be ruled out.[25] Santos-Silva and coleagues[26] reported a case of ONJ of the left posterior mandible that developed in a 61-year-old man with metastatic RCC treated with bevacizumab and temsirolimus. In 2013, Sato and colleagues[27] described a case of ONJ occurring in a patient with sigmoid colon cancer treated with the mFOLFOX6 regimen and bevacizumab. Surgical debridement of the necrotic bone and discontinuation of the bevacizumab resulted in resolution of the ONJ. Magremanne and colleagues[28] reported the case of a 49-year-old man with right temporal lobe glioblastoma treated with surgery and combined chemotherapy and radiation therapy; the radiation field did not include the jaws. The patient received a single dose of bevacizumab. There was no history of bisphosphonate therapy, but corticosteroids were part of the treatment regimen. One week after bevacizumab administration, tooth mobility with pain was noted in the left mandibular molar area. ONJ progressively worsened and an oral cutaneous communication developed. Lescaille and colleagues[29] studied a cohort of patients with cancer treated with ZA and identified 42 ONJ patients in the cohort, 10 of whom also had received bevacizumab. The mean duration of ZA treatment at the time of diagnosis of ONJ was 12.4 months in the bevacizumab/ZA group compared with 22.9 months in the 32 patients who received ZA only. In the bevacizumab/ZA group, 7 of 10 patients developed spontaneous ONJ. The conclusions, within the study limitations, suggested that patients receiving bevacizumab/ZA may develop spontaneous and earlier ONJ.[29] Bettini[30] reported a case of bevacizumab-related osteonecrosis of the mandible in a woman with non–small cell lung cancer. She was receiving multimodal chemotherapy containing bevacizumab, and there was no prior treatment with bisphosphonates. ONJ resolved after spontaneous bone sequestration a few months after cessation of bevacizumab.[30]

In 2009, Christodoulou and colleagues[13] reported a retrospective study analyzing the frequency of ONJ in those receiving combination bisphosphonates and antiangiogenic factors or bisphosphonates alone. The incidence of ONJ in patients receiving bisphosphonates with and without antiangiogenic agents was 16% and 1.1%, respectively.

Osteonecrosis of other anatomic sites other than the jaws has been reported in patients exposed to bevacizumab. Two cases of nasal septum perforation in patients on bevacizumab have been reported.[31,32] Osteonecrosis of the humeral head in a patient with non–small cell lung cancer receiving bevacizumab was reported by Kocywas and Cristea.[33] Bevacizumab-associated osteonecrosis of the wrist and knee was reported in 3 pediatric patients with recurrent central nervous system tumors.[34] None of the 3 patients had any exposure to a bisphosphonate, and 2 of them had received steroids.

MEDICATION-RELATED OSTEONECROSIS OF THE JAWS IN PATIENTS RECEIVING TYROSINE KINASE INHIBITORS, WITH AND WITHOUT ANTIRESORPTIVE EXPOSURE

To date, most cases of ONJ are related to the use of sunitinib and, to a lesser extent, sorafenib, both of which are TKIs with antiangiogenic effects. RCC is the primary malignancy treated with these drugs, and many (but not all) patients have received concomitant bisphosphonate treatment. The literature to date reflects mostly concomitant bisphosphonate use, but more recently many of these patients have been receiving concomitant denosumab. A few isolated cases of ONJ in patients receiving only a TKI have been reported.

Sunitinib (Sutent) is a small molecule that inhibits multiple receptor TKIs, such as those involved in tumor growth, pathologic angiogenesis, and metastatic progression of cancer. It inhibits many kinases including VEGF receptor 1 (VEGFR1), VEGFR2, and VEGFR3.[35] Sorafenib (Nexavar) is a kinase inhibitor that decreases tumor cell proliferation by inhibiting intracellular and cell surface kinases.[36]

Christodoulou and colleagues[13] reported ONJ in a 48-year-old man with RCC treated with sunitinib and ZA concurrently. Brunello and colleagues[37] reported a 59-year-old man with metastatic RCC treated with ZA who developed ONJ; sunitinib was subsequently added to his treatment regimen, after which the ONJ worsened with development of a cutaneous fistula. The condition improved on cessation of sunitinib but worsened on its resumption. The investigators hypothesized that the antiangiogenic activity of sunitinib amplified the inhibition of bone remodeling and antagonized mucosal healing.[37] Ayllon and colleagues[17] reported an RCC patient who was treated for hypercalcemia with ZA and was eventually placed on sunitinib, at which time ONJ developed; they postulated that the sunitinib may have been an activating factor in the onset of ONJ. Bozas and colleagues[38] reported a case of ONJ occurring after a single ZA infusion in a patient with metastatic RCC being treated with sunitinib. This patient had sunitinib-related mucositis before the development of ONJ. Concern was raised that with the increased concomitant use of sunitinib and bisphosphonates a possible synergistic effect may have occurred. Hoefert and Eufinger[39] reported 3 RCC patients with ONJ treated with sunitinib, 2 of whom received concurrent ZA and 1 ibandronate. Two patients with ONJ had sunitinib-related mucositis before ONJ. The third patient showed relapse of healed ONJ shortly after resumption of sunitinib.

Koch and colleagues[40] reported a 59-year-old man with RCC initially treated with interferon and vinblastine; after relapse, therapy was changed to sorafenib followed by sunitinib. One year later the patient developed ONJ, and there was no exposure to a bisphosphonate. Balmor and colleagues[41] reported a 63-year-old man with metastatic RCC who received sunitinib and monthly pamidronate, who developed postextraction ONJ of the maxilla and mandible. He underwent functional endoscopic sinus surgery for nasal bleeding for a nasal polyp and sleep apnea. Bisphosphonates were discontinued for 4 months before the surgery and sunitinib 2 weeks before the surgery. ONJ developed in the center of the hard palate with communication to the nasal cavity. The defect was obturated with a removable partial denture. Nicolatou-Galitis and colleagues[42] reported on 2 patients with oral complications related to sunitinib. One was a 19-year-old woman with RCC who was treated with cisplatin and sunitinib following recurrence of her tumor. She developed generalized gingival bleeding and the clinical features of necrotizing ulcerative gingivitis. Eventually necrotic bone was noted in the lingual mandible. Their second case was a 64-year-old woman with RCC who developed metastases and a new primary RCC in the contralateral kidney. Four years after starting sunitinib, she developed exposed bone of the lingual mandible. This patient had never received bisphosphonates. Sunitinib therapy was interrupted, and shortly thereafter a sequestrum developed. The area healed and the patient was placed on a reduced dose of sunitinib.[42] Fleissig and colleagues[43] reported a 58-year-old woman with recurrent RCC who developed ONJ 8 months after right mandibular third molar extraction. She was on sunitinib therapy, which was discontinued 14 days before the extraction and restarted 14 days after the extraction.

Beuselinck and colleagues[44] performed an institutional retrospective study on RCC patients with bone metastases treated with sunitinib or sorafenib over a 7-year period. Seventy-six patients were included: 49 treated with concomitant bisphosphonates and 27 with a TKI alone. Tumor response rates were significantly better in patients receiving bisphosphonates. The incidence of ONJ was 10% in patients treated with TKI and bisphosphonates. Agrillo and colleagues[45] reported 2 cases of ONJ in patients with RCC receiving sunitinib and the bisphosphonate ZA. The first patient was a 65-year-old man with metastatic RCC treated with sunitinib and ZA; he developed an oroantral communication with exposed bone. The second patient also had metastatic RCC; his treatment regimen consisted of sunitinib, but because of progression this was administered in association with temsirolimus. Subsequently, ONJ of the left mandible with cutaneous fistula was identified.[45] A retrospective study of 46 patients who received ZA and targeted therapy (TT) was performed by Smidt-Hansen and colleagues,[46] who examined 3 cohorts. Cohort A had 21 patients who received ZA and TT to prevent skeletal-related events, with no pretherapy oral and maxillofacial examination. Six patients (29%) developed ONJ, which was observed only in those receiving sunitinib and ZA. Cohort B had 16 patients who received TT and ZA for hypercalcemia, with no pretherapy oral and maxillofacial examination. No ONJ was observed in cohort B. Cohort C consisted of 9 patients who received TT and ZA along with pretherapy oral and maxillofacial examination. One patient (11%) developed ONJ during sunitinib and ZA treatment. It was concluded that combination ZA and TT was clinically beneficial but that ONJ may be exacerbated by concomitant ZA and sunitinib. Gulliet and colleagues[47] reported sorafenib-induced bilateral osteonecrosis of the femoral heads.

MEDICATION-RELATED OSTEONECROSIS OF THE JAWS IN PATIENTS RECEIVING MAMMALIAN TARGET OF RAPAMYCIN INHIBITORS WITH OR WITHOUT ANTIRESORPTIVE MEDICATIONS

mTOR is a key regulatory kinase of cell metabolism, growth, and differentiation. mTOR inhibitors directly affect this regulatory pathway. Several drugs classified as mTOR inhibitors are approved for use as an antineoplastic drug and for the prophylaxis of organ rejection in the transplant setting. Everolimus (Afinitor) has been approved for use in advanced hormone receptor–positive, HER2-negative breast cancer, advanced neuroendocrine tumors of pancreatic origin, advanced RCC, renal angiolyolipoma with tuberous sclerosis complex, and subependymal giant cell astrocytoma with tuberous sclerosis complex. Inhibition of mTOR by everolimus has an effect on cell proliferation and angiogenesis. Temsirolimus (Torisel) has been approved for use in advanced RCC, as it inhibits the activity of mTOR that controls cell division. The drug has an inhibitory effect on VEGF. Sirolimus (Rapamune) is indicated for the prophylaxis of organ rejection in patients receiving a renal transplant. Sirolimus inhibits cytokine-driven T-lymphocyte activation and proliferation.

Smidt-Hansen and colleagues,[46] reviewing several cohorts, referred to a case of a patient with metastatic RCC who developed ONJ while receiving everolimus as a second-line therapy. This patient had also received sunitinib and ZA, so the causative role of everolimus is unclear, as the sequencing of medication exposure and development of ONJ was not the focus of the study. These same investigators[46] also reported a patient who received temsirolimus as first-line therapy for metastatic RCC, but the patient who developed ONJ was also exposed to sunitinib and ZA.

MEDICATION-RELATED OSTEONECROSIS OF THE JAWS AND IMMUNOMODULATORY AGENTS WITH AN ANTIANGIOGENIC PROFILE

Thalidomide (Thalomid) and its analog, lenalidomide (Revlimid) alter the production of inflammatory cytokines including tumor necrosis factor α, interleukin (IL)-1, IL-6, IL-12, and the anti-inflammatory cytokine IL-10. Thalidomide, lenalidomide, and pomalidomide (Pomalyst) have also been shown to suppress angiogenesis. These drugs are frequently used in the treatment of multiple myeloma in combination with other medications with known risk factors for ONJ development, steroids such as prednisone and dexamethasone, and bisphosphonates.[48] Patients with multiple myeloma include a considerable percentage who develop ONJ.[48,49]

Tosi and colleagues,[50] in a letter to the editor, reported osteonecrosis of the jaws in patients newly diagnosed with multiple myeloma treated with ZA and thalidomide-dexamethasone. These investigators described how a limitation of the study was a shorter follow-up than in other such studies, but suggested that neither the antiangiogenic activity of thalidomide, nor impaired bone remodeling related to dexamethasone, nor severe immunosuppression induced by high-dose melphalan was an important risk factor for the development of ONJ.

SUMMARY

This review highlighted reported cases of ONJ in patients who received medications with antiangiogenic properties, with or without concomitant exposure to antiresorptive medications. Various medications such as the monoclonal inhibitor of angiogenesis (bevacizumab), TKIs such as sunitinib and sorafenib, the mTOR pathway inhibitors, and immunomodulatory agents such as thalidomide and its analogues are suspected to have a role in the pathogenesis of MRONJ.

REFERENCES

1. Arduino PG, Menegatti E, Scoletta M, et al. Vascular endothelial growth factor genetic polymorphisms an haplotypes in female patients with bisphosphonate-related osteonecrosis of the jaws. J Oral Pathol Med 2011;40:510–5.
2. Vincenzi B, Napolitano A, Zoccoli A, et al. Serum VEGF levels as predictive marker of bisphosphonate-related osteonecrosis of the jaw. J Hematol Oncol 2012;5:56.
3. Stressing V, Fournier PG, Bellahcene A, et al. Nitrogen-containing bisphosphonates can inhibit angiogenesis in vivo without the involvement of farnesyl pyrophosphate synthase. Bone 2011;48:259–66.
4. Misso G, Pornu M, Stoppacciaro A, et al. Evaluation of the in vitro and in vivo antiangiogenic effects of denosumab and zoledronic acid. Cancer Biol Ther 2012;13:1491–500.
5. Reid IR. Osteonecrosis of the jaw—who gets it, and why? Bone 2009;44:4–10.
6. Taylor KH, Middlefell LS, Mizen KD. Osteonecrosis of the jaws induced by anti-RANK ligand therapy. Br J Oral Maxillofac Surg 2010;48:221–3.
7. Kyrgidis A, Toulis KA. Denosumab-related osteonecrosis of the jaws. Osteoporos Int 2011;22:369–70.
8. Shim K, MacKenzie M, Winquist E. Chemotherapy-associated osteonecrosis in cancer patients with solid tumours. A systematic review. Drug Saf 2008; 31:359–71.
9. Sivolella S, Lumachi F, Stellini D, et al. Denosumab and anti-angiogenetic drug-related osteonecrosis of the jaw: an uncommon but potentially severe disease. Anticancer Res 2013;33:1793–7.
10. Jain RK, Duda DG, Clark JW, et al. Lessons from phase III clinical trials on anti-VEGF therapy for cancer. Nat Clin Pract Oncol 2006;3:24–40.
11. Lane HA, Wood JM, McSheehy PM, et al. mTOR inhibitor RAD001 (everolimus) has antiangiogenic/vascular properties distinct from a VEGFR tyrosine kinase inhibitor. Clin Cancer Res 2009;15:1612–22.
12. Yabu T, Tomimoto H, Taguchi Y, et al. Thalidomide-induced antiangiogenic action is mediated by ceramide through depletion of VEGF receptors, and is antagonized by shingosine-1-phosphate. Blood 2005;106:125–34.
13. Christodoulou C, Pervena A, Klouvas G. Combination of bisphosphonates and antiangiogenic factors induces osteonecrosis of the jaw more frequently than bisphosphonates alone. Oncology 2009;76:209–11.
14. Available at: http://www.rxlist.com/bevacizumab-drug/clinical-pharmacology.htm.
15. Estilo C, Fornier M, Farooki A, et al. Osteonecrosis of the jaw related to bevacizumab. J Clin Oncol 2008; 26:4037–43.
16. Greuter S, Schmid F, Ruhstaller T, et al. Bevacizumab-associated osteonecrosis of the jaw. Ann Oncol 2008;19:2091–2.
17. Ayllon J, Launay-Vacher V, Medioni J, et al. Osteonecrosis of the jaw under bisphosphonate and anti-angiogenic therapies: cumulative toxicity profile? Ann Oncol 2009;20:600–1.
18. Serra E, Paolantonio M, Spoto G, et al. Bevacizumab-related osteonecrosis of the jaw. Int J Immunopathol Pharmacol 2009;22:1121–3.
19. Guarneri V, Miles D, Robert N, et al. Bevacizumab and osteonecrosis of the jaw: incidence and association with bisphosphonate therapy in three large prospective trials in advanced breast cancer. Breast Cancer Res Treat 2010;122:181–8.

20. Francini F, Pascucci A, Francini F, et al. Osteonecrosis of the jaw in patients with cancer who received zoledronic acid and bevacizumab. J Am Dent Assoc 2011;142:506–13.

21. Ngamphaiboon N, Frustino J, Kossoff E, et al. Osteonecrosis of the jaw: dental outcomes in metastatic breast cancer patients treated with bisphosphonates with/without bevacizumab. Clin Breast Cancer 2011; 11:252–7.

22. Hopp R, Pucci J, Santos-Silva AR, et al. Osteonecrosis after administration of intravitreous bevacizumab. J Oral Maxillofac Surg 2012;70:632–5.

23. Disel U, Besen A, Er E, et al. Case report of bevacizumab-related osteonecrosis of the jaw: old problem, new culprit. Oral Oncol 2012;48:e2–3.

24. Brunamonti Binello P, Bandelloni R, Labanca M, et al. Osteonecrosis of the jaws and bevacizumab therapy: a case report. Int J Immunopathol Pharmacol 2012;25:789–91.

25. Katsenos S, Christophylakis C, Psathakis K. Osteonecrosis of the jaw in a patient with advanced non-small-cell lung cancer receiving bevacizumab. Arch Bronconeumol 2012;48:218–9.

26. Santos-Silva AR, Belizario Rosa GA, De Castro G Jr, et al. Osteonecrosis of the mandible associated with bevacizumab therapy. Oral Surg Oral Med Oral Pathol Oral Radiol 2013;115:e32–6.

27. Sato M, Ono F, Yamamura A, et al. A case of osteonecrosis of the jaw during treatment by bevacizumab for sigmoid colon cancer. Jpn J Gastroenterol 2013;110:655–9.

28. Magremanne M, Labon M, De Ceulaer J, et al. Unusual Bevacizumab-related complication of an oral infection. J Oral Maxillofac Surg 2013;71:53–5.

29. Lescaille G, Coudert A, Baaroun V, et al. Clinical study evaluating the effect of bevacizumab on the severity of zoledronic acid-related osteonecrosis of the jaw in cancer patients. Bone 2014;58:103–7.

30. Bettini G. Bevacizumab-related osteonecrosis of the mandible is a self-limiting disease process. BMJ Case Rep 2012.

31. Farkih MG, Lombardo JC. Bevacizumab-induced nasal septum perforation. Oncologist 2006;11:85–6.

32. Traina TA, Norton L, Drucker K, et al. Nasal Septum perforation in a bevacizumab-treated patient with metastatic breast cancer. Oncologist 2006;11:1070–1.

33. Koczywas M, Cristea MC. Osteonecrosis of the humeral head in a patient with non-small cell lung cancer receiving bevacizumab. J Thorac Oncol 2011;6: 1960–1.

34. Fangusaro J, Gururangan S, Jakacki R, et al. Bevacizumab-associated osteonecrosis of the wrist and knee in three pediatric patients with recurrent CNS tumors. J Clin Oncol 2012;33:e24–7.

35. Available at: http://www.rxlist.com/sutent-drug/clinical-pharmacology.htm.

36. Available at: http://www.rxlist.com/nexavar-drug/clinical-pharmacology.htm.

37. Brunello A, Saia G, Bedogni A, et al. Worsening of osteonecrosis of the jaw during treatment with sunitinib in a patient with metastatic renal cell carcinoma. Bone 2009;44:173–5.

38. Bozas G, Roy A, Ramasamy V, et al. Osteonecrosis of the jaw after a single bisphosphonate infusion in a patient with metastatic renal cancer treated with sunitinib. Onkologie 2010;33:321–3.

39. Hoefert A, Eufinger H. Sunitinib may raise the risk of bisphosphonate-related osteonecrosis of the jaw: presentation of three cases. Oral Surg Oral Med Oral Pathol Oral Radiol Endod 2010;110:463–9.

40. Koch FP, Walter C, Hansen T, et al. Osteonecrosis of the jaw related to sunitinib. Oral Maxillofac Surg 2011;15:63–6.

41. Balmor G, Yarom N, Weitzen R. Drug-Induced palate osteonecrosis following nasal surgery. Isr Med Assoc J 2012;14:193–4.

42. Nicolatou-Galitis O, Migkou M, Psyrri A, et al. Gingival bleeding and jaw bone necrosis in patients with metastatic renal cell carcinoma receiving sunitinib: report of 2 cases with clinical implications. Oral Surg Oral Med Oral Pathol Oral Radiol 2012;113:234–8.

43. Fleissig Y, Regev E, Lehman H. Sunitinib related osteonecrosis of jaw: a case report. Oral Maxillofac Surg 2012;113:e1–3.

44. Beuselinck B, Wolte P, Karadimou A, et al. Concomitant oral tyrosine kinase inhibitors and bisphosphonates in advanced renal cell carcinoma with bone metastases. Br J Cancer 2012;107:1665–71.

45. Agrillo A, Nastro Siniscalchi E, Facchini A, et al. Osteonecrosis of the jaws in patients assuming bisphosphonates and sunitinib: two case reports. Eur Rev Med Pharmacol Sci 2012;16:952–7.

46. Smidt-Hansen T, Folkmar T, Fode K, et al. Combination of zoledronic acid and targeted therapy is active but may induce osteonecrosis of the jaw in patients with metastatic renal cell carcinoma. J Oral Maxillofac Surg 2013;71:1532–40.

47. Gulliet M, Walter T, Scoazec JY, et al. Sorafenib-induced bilateral osteonecrosis of femoral heads. J Clin Oncol 2010;28:e14.

48. Otto S, Schreyer C, Hafner S, et al. Bisphosphonate-related osteonecrosis of the jaws—characteristics, risk factors, clinical features, localization and impact on oncology treatment. J Craniomaxillofac Surg 2012;40:303–9.

49. Badros A, Wekel D, Salama A. Osteonecrosis of the jaw in multiple myeloma patients: clinical features and risk factors. J Clin Oncol 2006;24:945–52.

50. Tosi P, Zamagni E, Cangini D, et al. Osteonecrosis of the jaws in newly diagnosed multiple myeloma patients treated with zolendronic acid and thalidomide-dexamethasone. Blood 2006;108:3951–2.

Antiresorptive Therapies for Osteoporosis

Stuart Weinerman, MD*, Gianina L. Usera, MD

KEYWORDS

- Antiresorptives • Bisphosphonates • Osteoporosis • Fracture • Osteonecrosis

KEY POINTS

- Antiresorptive agents are the most commonly used medications in osteoporosis.
- The end result of antiresorptive agent use is a net decrease of bone turnover and an increase in bone mineralization.
- Bone turnover consists of a stepwise process of resorption and formation of bone. When the balance favors resorption, a net loss in bone strength and quality is seen.
- Although rare, one of the main concerns when treating patients with bisphosphonates and monoclonal antibodies against receptor activator of nuclear factor-κB ligand is osteonecrosis of the jaw.

Bones have a versatile nature, being stiff enough to resist deformation, and flexible enough to absorb energy by deforming. Made up of type I collagen and calcium hydroxyapatite crystals, they achieve these characteristics by being 60% mineralized.[1] Depending on their structure and composition, bones are able to lengthen, shorten, and widen to allow for loading and movement. Long bones serve as levers, whereas the vertebral bodies retain a spring action. They adapt through modeling and remodeling, undergoing reconstruction by the bone multicellular unit. This unit is made up of osteoclasts and osteoblasts that work in symphony to resorb and replace bone that has sustained an insult. These cells move in waves over microcracks and surrounding matrix, breaking down damaged areas and depositing new lamellar bone in its place (**Fig. 1**). In this process, osteoclasts are always followed by osteoblasts. It is through this mechanism that the peak strength of a bone is achieved during the formative years, and then maintained in adulthood. At any time, there will be bone that was resorbed but not yet replaced, and this is known as the remodeling space. Depending on what stage in life one is in, the balance of formation and resorption will vary. During growth, the balance is positive with bone formation in the forefront, whereas during aging the balance tips negatively when the remodeling rate increases (**Fig. 2**).[2]

Osteoporosis is a disorder of compromised bone strength resulting in an increased risk of fracture. It is estimated that 55% of people over 50 years old have osteoporosis. In the United States, this comes out to about 10 million people with osteoporosis and 34 million with osteopenia.[3] In 2002, it is estimated that osteoporosis cost the economy 18 billion with hospital and nursing home admissions. This is not surprising; 1 in 5 fracture patients ends up in nursing homes.[4] Putting osteoporosis into perspective, women over 50 years of age have a lifetime risk of osteoporosis of 50% versus a 12% risk of developing breast cancer, and men over 50 years of age have a 20% lifetime risk of osteoporosis versus a 17% risk of prostate cancer.[5] Some risk factors for developing osteoporosis include low bone mineral density (BMD), age greater than 50 years, hormone

The authors have no financial or commercial conflicts of interest to disclose.
Division of Endocrinology & Diabetes, Department of Medicine, Hofstra North Shore-LIJ School of Medicine, 865 Northern Boulevard, Suite 203, Great Neck, New York 11021, USA
* Corresponding author.
E-mail address: sweinerm@nshs.edu

Oral Maxillofacial Surg Clin N Am 27 (2015) 555–560
http://dx.doi.org/10.1016/j.coms.2015.07.001
1042-3699/15/$ – see front matter © 2015 Elsevier Inc. All rights reserved.

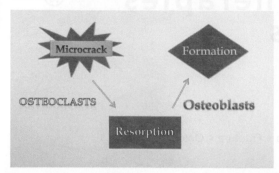

Fig. 1. Bone remodeling.

Table 1
Antiresorptives & fracture efficacy

Drugs	Vertebral	Nonvertebral	Hip
Alendronate	X	X	X
Ibandronate	X	None	None
Risedronate	X	X	X
Zoledronic Acid	X	X	X
Denosumab	X	X	X
SERMs*	X	None	None
Estrogen	X	X	X
Calcitonin	X	None	None

* Selective estrogen receptor modulators.

deficiency, smoking, certain medications such as corticosteroids or chemotherapy, and excessive alcohol use. It is a huge public health problem, especially because 80% of high-risk patients with 1 osteoporotic fracture are neither identified nor treated.[2] As mentioned, there exists a negative balance in bone resorption and formation, with resulting bone loss beginning around ages 18 to 30. Antiresorptive medications used for treatment of osteoporosis reduce the rate of remodeling and therefore promote completion of bone formation in remodeling sites present before commencement of treatment.

Antiresorptive medications and anabolic agents comprise the 2 main treatment options for osteoporosis. There are currently 5 classes of antiresorptive agents approved for use: bisphosphonates, monoclonal antibodies against receptor activator of nuclear factor-κB ligand (RANKL), selective estrogen receptor modulators (SERMs), estrogens, and calcitonin (**Table 1**).[6] There is abundant evidence demonstrating the efficacy of antiresorptives in preventing fractures, especially in postmenopausal women. We currently have only 1 anabolic therapeutic agent, teriparatide, which is usually reserved for patients with severe osteoporosis or

at a high risk of fracture. For the purposes of this article, we focus on the antiresorptive medications.

Bisphosphonates are the most widely used class of osteoporosis treatments. The compounds are synthetic analogs of inorganic pyrophosphate, where the central oxygen is replaced by a carbon atom. The differences between molecules are owing to variable side chains off the central molecule. Adding a hydroxyl group to the central carbon enhances the affinity to calcium crystals. The addition of a nitrogen atom to the other side chain attached to the central carbon has significant impact on decreasing bone resorption. The first molecule, etidronate, was initially designed to soften toward order for industrial purposes. The first biological use of etidronate began in the 1960s as a treatment of decreasing unwanted calcium deposition is soft tissues, namely, heterotopic ossification.[7] Further research suggested that this drug would also impair osteoclast mediated bone resorption. The initial theory was that this was owing to stabilization of hydroxyapatite crystals. Further investigation showed that this was a direct effect on osteoclast function. Initial compounds, which did not have a nitrogen atom attached to the central carbon, seemed to be nonspecific inhibitors at the adenosine triphosphate function and caused cell apoptosis. Compounds that contained a nitrogen atom as part of the central side were eventually found to have a very specific effect of inhibition of farnesyl pyrophosphate synthase, an enzyme related to the hydroxymethylglutaryl–mevalonic cholesterol synthesis pathway. Inhibition of this enzyme seems to affect prenylation, or binding to fat chains, of small intracellular regulatory proteins, which decreases function of the osteoclasts. There is a very good correlation between the potency of the aminobisphosphonates in vitro on inhibition of this enzyme and the antiresorptive efficacy of the compounds.

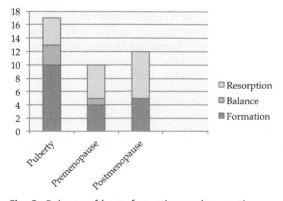

Fig. 2. Balance of bone formation and resorption.

The compounds share similar pharmacokinetics. The intestinal absorption of the bisphosphonates is poor, generally in the range of 0.5%, and this is why these drugs have to be given on an empty stomach (except for Atelvia, a specially coated form of risedronate). The drugs are rapidly cleared from the blood and either taken up into the skeleton, targeting areas of high bone remodeling, or excreted in the urine. The drugs have a very long half-life in bone, which may have impact for long-term adverse effects as well as the possibility of drug holidays.

The primary effect is to decrease osteoclast function and bone resorption. This translates into a slower rate of bone remodeling, allowing the osteoblasts to fill in bone remodeling spaces (**Fig. 3**). There is a tight coupling of osteoclast and osteoblastic activity whereby reducing osteoclastic activity eventually turns down osteoblastic activity as well. Newer compounds such as odanocatib have the potential for uncoupling this process, decreasing bone resorption without affecting bone formation.

The human monoclonal antibody denosumab is a newer type of medication for the treatment of osteoporosis. This drug works by inhibiting RANKL. RANKL is a protein that is the primary mediator of osteoclast activity, and necessary for osteoclast formation. Denosumab binds with high affinity to it, resulting in a reduction of osteoblast number and function. It is very effective at improving BMD and reducing the risk of hip, vertebral, and nonvertebral fractures. The main 2 concerns of side effects are similar to bisphosphonates—osteonecrosis of the jaw and atypical femur fractures. Hypocalcaemia is another side effect to monitor, and a blood test before each dose should be obtained.

Estrogens were once the first-line therapy for prevention of fractures in postmenopausal women. Menopause, a state of estrogen deficiency, is known to have increased rates of bone remodeling, which have been associated to higher risk of fracture. Estrogens suppress bone resorption by blocking cytokine activation signals of osteoclasts. In the Women's Health Initiative study, 16,608 postmenopausal women were treated with 0.625 mg estrogen plus 2.5 mg medroxyprogesterone daily, which resulted in 34% reduction of vertebral and hip fractures. The Women's Health Initiative trials also showed an increased risk of women treated with estrogen to developing breast cancer, coronary artery disease, and thromboembolic events.[8] For these reasons, it is only used to treat menopausal symptoms presently.

SERMs inhibit bone resorption through the same mechanism as estrogens. These drugs can be used for the prevention and treatment of postmenopausal osteoporosis, although they are generally less effective than bisphosphonates. They act like estrogen agonists at bone and as estrogen antagonists at breast. Owing to this dual action, this class of medications also reduces the risk of invasive breast cancer in women who are at high risk. Patients treated with SERMs, like those on estrogen, are at an increased risk of developing thromboembolic events.[9,10]

Calcitonin is a 32-amino acid endogenous peptide hormone with only a modest reduction in bone turnover. It is the least potent agent and generally not used. It binds to osteoclasts through high-affinity receptors, and also produces an analgesic effect on painful vertebral fractures. Because the most popular formulation of this medicine is a nasal spray, some of the more common side effects are at the site of administration, like sneezing and rhinitis.[6]

There have been many large, randomized, controlled trials proving fracture efficacy with these drugs. Once a drug has been proven to reduce fractures, the US Food and Drug Administration (FDA) allows "bridging" studies, using bone density as endpoint, for other populations. For example, if the studies in postmenopausal women proved fracture protection, studies in men or patients on glucocorticoids were much smaller, based on bone density results and not powered for fractures.

One of the first studies to look at one of the bisphosphonates, alendronate, was the Fracture Intervention Trial (FIT) in 1996. This randomized, double-blind, placebo-controlled trial followed for 36 months 2027 women ages 55 to 81 that were assigned to receive either placebo or alendronate. The initial dose of alendronate was 5 mg/d for the first 24 months, and then subsequently increased to 10 mg/d for the remaining 12 months. The primary endpoints were new vertebral fractures

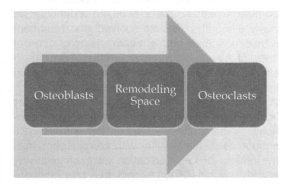

Fig. 3. Remodeling space.

and risk of new clinical fractures. Radiographs of the spine were done at 24 and 36 months. The results of the study showed that the group treated with alendronate had a decrease in the incidence of new morphometric fractures (8% new in treatment group vs 15% in placebo group). The secondary endpoint of new clinical fractures was also decreased in the treatment arm (13.6% vs 18.2% in the placebo group).[11] Following the results of this study, the same group of researchers in 1998 looked at whether there was also a decrease in the risk of fracture in women with low BMD but no history of prior fractures. This arm of the FIT study compared treatment with alendronate versus placebo for 4 years, with the main endpoint being a decrease in the risk of clinical and vertebral fractures. A total of 8704 women were enrolled, and about one-half were randomized to the treatment arm, and the other one-half to placebo. The dose of the alendronate group was 5 mg/d for the first 2 years followed by 10 mg/d for the remainder of the study. The intervention group showed a 36% decrease of clinical fractures in women with baseline osteoporosis, but no significant decrease in women with higher baseline BMD. Alendronate also reduced radiographic vertebral fractures by 44%.[12] Essentially, what the FIT and FLEX trials showed was that alendronate is effective for patients with osteoporosis in decreasing the risk of fracture and increasing BMD.

Another important bisphosphonate trial looks at the effect of risedronate in women with postmenopausal osteoporosis. This was the Vertebral Efficacy With Risedronate Therapy (VERT) Study Group, published in 1999. When this trial was commenced, risedronate was known to be effective in Paget disease of bone and other metabolic bone disorders. The goal of the trial was to test the efficacy and safety of daily treatment with risedronate in decreasing the risk of vertebral and other fractures in postmenopausal women with known osteoporosis. This randomized, double-blind, placebo-controlled trial included 2458 women younger than 85 years old with history of at least 1 vertebral fracture. The intervention group was assigned either 2.5 or 5 mg/d of risedronate. The main outcome measures were incidence of new vertebral fractures and nonvertebral fractures seen radiographically, or increase of BMD. After 1 year, the 2.5 mg/d dose group was discontinued, whereas the 5 mg/d dose and placebo arms completed total of 3 years. The 5 mg/d dose arm showed a 41% decrease in the incidence of new vertebral fractures, and a significant increase in BMD. The safety profile was found to be similar to that of the placebo group.[13] Years

later, when a monthly dosing formulation of risedronate was manufactured, a study was done to examine the efficacy and safety of this treatment option. This randomized, double-blind trial lasted 2 years and enrolled 1094 participants. There were 2 treatment arms, one on 5 mg/d dosing and the other on 150 mg monthly. Mean percent change in lumbar spine BMD was 3.4% and 3.5%, respectively. In conclusion, the monthly dosing was similar in efficacy and safety as the daily dosing.[14]

Ibandronate, another bisphosphonate, was studied in 2004 with a randomized, double-blind, placebo-controlled, parallel-group study that enrolled 2946 postmenopausal women. There were 3 groups, consisting of placebo, 2.5 mg/d and intermittently 20 mg every other day for 12 doses every 3 months. The study duration was 3 years, and it found that the rate of new vertebral fractures was significantly reduced in patients receiving oral daily (4.7%) and intermittent ibandronate (4.9%), relative to placebo (9.6%).[15]

Zoledronic acid, a bisphosphonate with an intravenous formulation, was studied in a 3-year, double-blind, placebo-controlled trial in 2007. A total of 7765 patients were enrolled and randomized to receive either a single 15-minute infusion of zoledronic acid 5 mg dose or placebo at baseline, 12 months, and 24 months. They were followed until 36 months. Main outcome measures were new vertebral fracture and hip fracture. Secondary outcome measures included BMD, bone turnover markers, and safety outcomes. The results showed a reduced risk of morphometric vertebral fracture by 70%, a reduced risk of hip fracture by 41%, and that the effect on biochemical markers was similar to those reported for oral bisphosphonates.[16]

Last, the human monoclonal antibody to the RANKL, denosumab, was studied in the FREEDOM trial in 2009. This 3-year, placebo-controlled, randomized trial included postmenopausal women aged 60 to 90 years old. There were a total of 7868 participants enrolled, and randomized to either placebo or 60 mg of denosumab every 6 months. Results showed that treatment with denosumab had a relative risk reduction of 68% of new radiographic vertebral fractures. It also was found to relatively reduce the risk of hip fractures by 40% and nonvertebral fractures by 20%. In addition, denosumab use did not delay fracture healing or contribute to other complications. A particularity of treatment with RANKL antibodies is that, unlike with bisphosphonates, the effects of the medication wear off relatively quickly, within 6 to 12 months after discontinuation. Some side effects noted were local symptoms of swelling and dermatitis.[17] However, with the higher doses used for treatment of patients with bone metastasis, there is a greater risk of developing osteonecrosis of the jaw.

There is a growing body of evidence that treating patients with bisphosphonates for longer than 10 years puts these patients at a higher risk of developing side effects of osteonecrosis of the jaw and atypical femur fractures.[18] This has lead to the concept of "drug holiday," or stopping therapy after 3 to 5 years, as recommended by the FDA advisory September 2011. There are 2 bases to support this approach. This class of drugs has a long-term half-life in bone, and the antiresorptive effects remain potent even off therapy. This treatment strategy does not apply to any other class of therapy, such as estrogen or denosumab; studies have shown rapid bone loss upon stopping therapy. The second basis is that stopping or holding therapy will reduce adverse effects.

Two major trials compared shorter versus long-term therapy. After the completion of the original alendronate study, it was extended for 5 more years to look at safety and efficacy of longer duration of treatment with alendronate. This is known as the Long-term Experience with Alendronate FIT Long-term Extension (FLEX) study. A total of 1099 participants were enrolled, with the intervention group given either 5 or 10 mg/d doses of alendronate. Clinical vertebral fractures were reduced by 55% overall in treatment group but did not reduce risk of nonvertebral fractures or morphometric vertebral fractures. Nonvertebral fractures were reduced by 50% in continuing women with osteoporosis as measured at femoral neck at the start of FLEX, but not in those with higher BMD or patients with low bone density and prevalent vertebral fractures.[19] This inconsistency in this post hoc analysis led the FDA advisory committee to reject the fracture claims.

The second major extension trial evaluated 3 versus 6 years of intravenous zoledronate. This trial showed no difference in clinical fractures, but a small decrease in morphometric vertebral fractures, the opposite of the FLEX spine results. Neither trial was powered to evaluate an effect of drug holiday on osteonecrosis of the jaw or atypical femur fractures.

An epidemiologic study from Sweden did show that drug cessation was associated with an early 70% reduction in atypical fractures.[20] Bisphosphonate drug holidays have become the standard approach in the management of osteoporosis, but remain controversial. Many experts have recommended continuing therapy in patients with a persistent high risk of fracture.

REFERENCES

1. Seeman E, Delmas PD. Bone quality — the material and structural basis of bone strength and fragility. N Engl J Med 2006;354(21):2250–61.
2. Primer on the metabolic bone diseases and disorders of mineral metabolism. In: Rosen CJ, editor. 8th edition. Wiley-Blackwell; 2013.
3. Available at: NOF.org/osteoporosis/diseasefacts. Accessed February, 2015.
4. Available at: iofbonehealth.org/facts-statistics. Accessed February, 2015.
5. Available at: cancer.gov/cancertopics/factsheet/detection/probability-breast-cancer. Accessed February, 2015.
6. Chen JS, Sambrook PN. Antiresorptive therapies for osteoporosis: a clinical overview. Nat Rev 2011;8: 81–91.
7. Rosen CJ. A tale of two worlds in prescribing etidronate for osteoporosis. Lancet 1997;350(9088):1340.
8. Available at: nhlbi.nih.gov/whi/. Accessed February, 2015.
9. Cummings SR, Eckert S, Krueger KA, et al. The effect of raloxifene on risk of breast cancer in postmenopausal women: results from the MORE randomized trial. Multiple outcomes of raloxifene evaluation. JAMA 1999;281(23):2189–97.
10. Ettinger B, Black DM, Mitlak BH, et al. Reduction of vertebral fracture risk in postmenopausal women with osteoporosis treated with raloxifene: results from a 3-year randomized clinical trial. Multiple outcomes of raloxifene evaluation (MORE) investigators. JAMA 1999;282(7):637–45.
11. Black DM, Cummings SR, Karpf DB, et al. Randomized trial of effect of alendronate on risk of fracture in women with existing vertebral fractures. Fracture Intervention Trial Research Group. Lancet 1996; 348(9041):1535–41.
12. Cummings SR, Black DM, Thompson DE, et al. Effect of alendronate on risk of fracture in women with low bone density but without vertebral fractures: results from the Fracture Intervention Trial. JAMA 1998;280(24):2077–82.
13. Harris ST, Watts NB, Genant HK, et al. Effects of risedronate treatment on vertebral and nonvertebral fractures in women with postmenopausal osteoporosis: a randomized controlled trial. Vertebral Efficacy with Risedronate Therapy (VERT) Study Group. JAMA 1999;282(14):1344–52.
14. Delmas PD, McClung MR, Zanchetta JR, et al. Efficacy and safety of risedronate 150 mg a month in treatment of postmenopausal osteoporosis. Bone 2008;42(1):36–42.
15. Chestnut C, Skag A, Christiansen C, et al. Effects of oral ibandronate administered daily or intermittently on fracture risk in postmenopausal osteoporosis. J Bone Miner Res 2004;19(8):1241–9.

16. Black DM, Delmas PD, Eastell R, et al. Once-yearly zoledronic acid for treatment of postmeno-pausal osteoporosis. N Engl J Med 2007;356: 1809–22.

17. Cummings SR, San Martin J, McClung MR, et al, FREEDOM Trial. Denosumab for prevention of frac-tures in postmenopausal women with osteoporosis. N Engl J Med 2009;361(8):756–65.

18. Watts NB, Diab D. Efficacy of continued alendronate for fractures in women with and without prevalent vertebral fracture: the FLEX trial. J Clin Endocrinol Metab 2010;95(4):1555–65.

19. Schwartz AV, Bauer DC, Cummings SR, et al. Effi-cacy of continued alendronate for fractures in women with and without prevalent vertebral frac-ture: the FLEX trial. J Bone Miner Res 2010;25: 976–82.

20. Schilcher J, Michaëlsson K, Aspenberg P, et al. Bisphosphonate use and atypical fractures of the femoral shaft. N Engl J Med 2011;364:1728–37.

Antiresorptive Therapies for the Treatment of Malignant Osteolytic Bone Disease

Bhoomi Mehrotra, MD

KEYWORDS

- Antiresorptive therapy • Bisphosphonate
- Receptor activator of nuclear factor κB ligand (RANKL) inhibitor (denosumab) • Zoledronic acid
- Pamidronate • Malignant bone disease • Osteolytic bone disease

KEY POINTS

- Antiresorptive therapies, such as bisphosphonates and the receptor activator of nuclear factor κB ligand (RANKL) inhibitor (denosumab), are an established standard of care in the management of malignant osteolytic bone disease. They have been shown to improve the quality of life of patients with cancer who have advanced bony disease and to attenuate the negative effects of antiandrogens on bone health in patients with prostate cancer and the effects of aromatase inhibitors in the management of breast cancer.
- Bisphosphonates seem to have a role in improving survival in patients with multiple myeloma and may have a role in improving disease-free survival in the adjuvant therapy for hormone sensitive breast cancer.
- Current laboratory investigations to understand their mechanism of action and clinical studies to optimize their indications, dosage schedule, and duration of therapy are ongoing. These will help elucidate their evolving role in the management of patients with malignant disease.

INTRODUCTION

Oral bisphosphonate therapy has proven efficacy in the management of osteoporosis. Numerous more potent aminobisphosphonates, which are administered intravenously, such as pamidronate and zoledronic acid, are known to irreversibly bind to the bony matrix and make them resistant to the osteolytic activity of malignant cells. Initial clinical trials evaluated the role of aminobisphosphonates in inhibiting osteolytic activity and thereby controlling hypercalcemia of malignancy. Subsequent clinical trials evaluated the role of intravenous bisphosphonates in reducing pain related to skeletal lesions, delaying the time to skeletal-related events, reducing the incidence of compression fractures, reducing the need for orthopedic manipulations, reducing the need for radiation therapy, and improving the quality of life. Such trials initially focused on predominantly malignant diseases that led to osteolytic bony metastasis such as breast cancer, renal cell cancer, and multiple myeloma. Subsequent trials focused on malignant bone disease, even those of osteoblastic nature such as typically seen in metastatic prostate cancer. Zoledronic acid therapy was shown to be superior to pamidronate therapy in all malignant causes of bony disease except in multiple myeloma in which both agents were equally efficacious. Subsequent discovery

Department of Medicine, Cancer Institute at St. Francis Hospital, The Heart Center, 100 Port Washington Boulevard, Roslyn, NY 11576, USA
E-mail address: bhoomi.mehrotra@chsli.org

Oral Maxillofacial Surg Clin N Am 27 (2015) 561–566
http://dx.doi.org/10.1016/j.coms.2015.07.002
1042-3699/15/$ – see front matter © 2015 Elsevier Inc. All rights reserved.

of receptor activator of nuclear factor κB ligand (RANKL) inhibitor (denosumab), which is a fully humanized antibody against RANKL that inhibits osteoclast function and consequent bone resorption has proven to be equally or more efficacious than aminobisphosphonates in the management of solid tumor-related metastatic bone disease. However, denosumab therapy is inferior to bisphosphonate therapy in the treatment of multiple myeloma-related bone disease.

Several trials have explored the role of antiresorptive therapy in the prevention of osteolytic bone disease during the natural history of a patient afflicted with advanced solid tumors. However, thus far, these data remain elusive. Bisphosphonate therapies have also been evaluated as adjuvant therapy in the management of early stage primary breast cancer. There are conflicting data regarding their role in impacting overall survival. However, there seems to be benefit from the addition of zoledronic acid to adjuvant endocrine therapy in premenopausal women with estrogen-responsive early breast cancer when evaluated for disease-free survival. In postmenopausal women, there seems to be a clear benefit in terms of disease-free survival of adjuvant bisphosphonates (oral or intravenous). In addition, adjuvant denosumab has been shown to abrogate aromatase inhibitor therapy-related adverse effects on the bone by significantly delaying the time to first clinical fracture.

Antiresorptive therapies have, therefore, become a standard part of the armamentarium of anticancer therapies as supportive and complementary agents in individuals with advanced disease. They are also now being evaluated in the adjuvant setting of oncologic managements and as preventative agents before the development

of clinically symptomatic bony disease. This article focuses primarily on the 3 parenteral antiresorptive agents approved by the Food and Drug Administration (FDA) (**Table 1**) in the United States for the management of malignant bone disease: pamidronate, zoledronic acid, and denosumab.

PAMIDRONATE

Pamidronate disodium is an aminobisphosphonate that is indicated in the treatment of tumor-induced hypercalcemia, bone metastases, multiple myeloma, and Paget disease of the bone. It is a potent inhibitor of osteoclastic bone resorption in that it inhibits access of osteoclast precursors onto bone and their subsequent transformation into mature, resorbing osteoclasts.[1] It has a strong affinity for calcified tissues and it is almost exclusively eliminated by renal excretion.

Pamidronate disodium was initially evaluated in the treatment of cancer-related hypercalcemia. In a landmark trial by Gucalp and colleagues,[2] a single infusion of 60 mg of pamidronate was more effective than etidronate in the treatment of cancer-related hypercalcemia. After its role was proven in the management of hypercalcemia of malignancy, it was further evaluated in the management of bone metastases in several solid tumors and multiple myeloma. Berenson and colleagues[3] showed that monthly infusions of pamidronate provide significant protection against skeletal complications and improvement in the quality of life in subjects with stage III multiple myeloma. Subjects with stage III multiple myeloma and at least one lytic lesion received either placebo or 90 mg of pamidronate as a 4-hour intravenous infusion given every 4 weeks for 9 cycles in addition to antimyeloma therapy. Skeletal events

Table 1
Antiresorptive agents approved by the Food and Drug Administration in the United States

Agents	Oncologic Indications
Pamidronate	• Tumor-induced hypercalcemia • Predominantly lytic metastases from solid tumors and multiple myeloma
Zoledronic acid	• Hypercalcemia of malignancy • Patients with multiple myeloma and patients with documented bone metastases from solid tumors (in conjunction with standard antineoplastic therapy) • Patients with prostate cancer who have progressive disease after treatment with at least one hormonal therapy
Denosumab[a]	• Prevention of skeletal-related events in patients with bone metastases from solid tumors • Treatment of giant cell tumor of bone that is unresectable • Treatment of hypercalcemia of malignancy refractory to bisphosphonate therapy

[a] Denosumab is not indicated for the prevention of skeletal-related events in patients with multiple myeloma.

(pathologic fracture, irradiation of or surgery on bone, and spinal cord compression), hypercalcemia, bone pain, analgesic use, performance status, and quality of life were assessed. Among 392 treated subjects, the proportion of subjects who had any skeletal events was significantly lower in the pamidronate group (24%) than in the placebo group (41%). Subjects who received pamidronate also had significant decreases in bone pain and maintained their performance status and quality of life.

Efficacy of pamidronate in reducing skeletal complications in subjects with breast cancer and lytic bone metastases was evaluated by Hortobagyi and colleagues.[4] Women with stage IV breast cancer who were receiving chemotherapy and had at least one lytic bone lesion were given either placebo or pamidronate infusions monthly for 12 cycles. The median time to the occurrence of the first skeletal complication was greater in the pamidronate group than in the placebo. As was seen in the multiple myeloma trial, the proportion of subjects in whom skeletal complication occurred was also lower in the pamidronate group compared with the placebo. There was also significantly less increase in bone pain and deterioration of performance status in the pamidronate group than in the placebo group. In both trials, pamidronate was well tolerated. Intravenous administration is commonly associated with transient fever and flu-like symptoms that resolve spontaneously. Other common adverse effects included gastrointestinal symptoms of nausea, vomiting, anorexia, diarrhea, constipation, skin rash, transient bone pain, arthralgia, myalgia, generalized pain, and reactions at the infusion site. Reported uncommon adverse effects include orbital inflammation, osteonecrosis of the jaw, atypical subtrochanteric and diaphyseal femoral fractures, renal tubular disorders, and focal segmental glomerulosclerosis.

ZOLEDRONIC ACID (ZOLEDRONATE)

Zoledronic acid (zoledronate) is a bisphosphonic acid that is a potent inhibitor of osteoclastic bone resorption. Although the precise antiresorptive mechanism is not completely understood, in vitro, zoledronic acid inhibits osteoclastic activity and induces osteoclast apoptosis.[5] By avidly binding to bony matrix, zoledronic acid inhibits the osteoclastic resorption of mineralized bone and cartilage. Zoledronic acid is indicated in the treatment of hypercalcemia of malignancy, management of bone metastases from solid tumors, multiple myeloma, and in patients being treated concurrently with standard antineoplastic therapy.

It is also indicated in the management of patients with advanced hormone refractory prostate cancer.

Zoledronic acid is superior to pamidronate in the treatment of hypercalcemia of malignancy. A pooled analysis of two randomized controlled clinical trials by Major and colleagues[6] evaluated 287 subjects with moderate to severe hypercalcemia of malignancy who were treated either with a single dose of zoledronic acid or pamidronate. Zoledronic acid was shown to be superior to pamidronate because normalization of serum calcium occurred in 50% of subjects treated with zoledronic acid and in only 33.3% of pamidronate-treated subjects by day 4. The median duration of complete response also favored zoledronic acid compared with pamidronate.

Zoledronic acid, in addition to endocrine therapy, has been evaluated as adjuvant therapy for premenopausal women with estrogen-responsive early breast cancer. For the Austrian Breast and Colorectal Cancer Study Group (ABCSG) trial 12, Gnant and colleagues[7] examined the effect of zoledronic acid in combination with antiestrogen therapies in premenopausal women with endocrine-responsive early breast cancer. The addition of zoledronic acid to endocrine therapy, compared with endocrine therapy without zoledronic acid, resulted in an absolute reduction of 3.2% points and a relative reduction of 35% in the risk of disease progression. However, the addition of zoledronic acid did not significantly reduce the risk of death.

For the Adjuvant Zoledronic Acid to Reduce Recurrence (AZURE) trial, Coleman and colleagues[8] evaluated the role of zoledronic acid in addition to standard adjuvant systemic therapy for breast cancer. At a median follow-up of 59 months, there was no significant difference with the rate of disease-free survival in the zoledronic acid group versus the control group.

A multi-institutional (SWOG (South West Oncology Group)/Alliance/ECOG (Eastern Cooperative Oncology Group)-ACRIN (American College of Radiology Imaging Network)/NCIC (National Cancer Institute of Canada) Clinical Trials Group/NRG Oncology study S0307) phase III trial of bisphosphonates as adjuvant therapy in the management of primary breast cancer[9] was recently presented at the 2015 American Society of Clinical Oncology annual meeting. Subjects with stage I to III breast cancer receiving adjuvant systemic therapy were randomized to receive 3 years of clodronate, ibandronate, or zoledronic acid. The primary endpoint was disease-free survival. The primary outcome of the trial (ie, disease-free survival) did not differ across the arms. Overall survival was

93% in all 3 arms. This study did not find evidence of differences in efficacy by type of bisphosphonate used. Therefore, the role of zoledronic acid in the adjuvant management of breast cancer remains unclear at this time.

Zoledronic acid is known to decrease the risk for skeletal-related events in men with castrate-resistant prostate cancer but its role earlier in the natural history of prostate cancer is unclear. A recent phase III trial evaluated the efficacy and safety of earlier treatment with zoledronic acid in men with castration-sensitive metastatic prostate cancer. Men with castration-sensitive prostate cancer and bone metastases whose androgen deprivation therapy was initiated within 6 months of study entry were randomized to receive zoledronic acid (4 mg intravenously every 4 weeks) or a placebo. Early zoledronic acid was not associated with increased time to first skeletal-related event. Overall survival was also similar between the groups.[10]

The efficacy and safety of zoledronic acid has also been evaluated in subjects with bone metastases secondary to solid tumors other than breast or prostate cancer. In a study of 773 such cases, subjects were randomized to receive zoledronic acid or placebo every 3 weeks for 9 months with concomitant antineoplastic therapy. Subjects receiving zoledronic acid had significantly increased time to a first skeletal event and significantly reduced the risk of developing the skeletal events.[11]

A recent randomized phase III trial conducted by CALGB (Cancer and Leukemia Group) 70604[12] has evaluated standard dosing versus longer interval dosing of zoledronic acid in metastatic cancer. In this randomized trial, 1822 subjects with breast, prostate, myeloma, and other cancers were randomized to receive either zoledronic acid monthly or every 3 months for 24 months. The 2-year cumulative incidence of skeletal-related events was similar in both groups. The risk of osteonecrosis of the jaw was reduced by 50% in the group administered to every 3 months (18 of 911 subjects in the every month group vs 9 of 911 in the every 3 month group). Further analysis of this study's results is ongoing. The optimal duration and frequency of zoledronic acid administration remains unclear.

The most common adverse event related to the infusion of zoledronic acid are infusion-related flu-like symptoms that are typically self-remitting, nausea, fatigue, anemia, bone pain, constipation, fever, vomiting, and dyspnea. Zoledronic acid is excreted intact primarily via the kidney and renal adverse reactions may be greater in patients with impaired renal function. The dosing of zoledronic acid is adjusted before each administration based on the creatinine clearance and dose modifications have been well-established and reported in the package insert.[5] Other uncommon side effects include osteonecrosis of the jaw, atypical subtrochanteric and diaphyseal femoral fractures, musculoskeletal pain, and hypocalcemia. As discussed previously, an acute phase reaction that occurs within 3 days after zoledronic acid administration is often noted with symptoms including fevers, fatigue, bone pain, and flu-like symptomatology. These symptoms typically resolve spontaneously within a few days. Rare cases of uveitis, scleritis, episcleritis, conjunctivitis, and orbital inflammation have been reported during postmarketing use. To reduce the risk of renal toxicity, it is recommended that the dose of zoledronic acid of 4 mg be administered as an intravenous infusion over 15 minutes.

In several randomized trials comparing zoledronic acid with pamidronate in the management of multiple myeloma, zoledronic acid seems to be noninferior to pamidronate therapy. It has been hypothesized that bisphosphonates may have an antimyeloma effect. In the Medical Research Council Myeloma IX trial, zoledronic acid administration, in addition to standard antimyeloma therapy, improved overall survival and progression-free survival when evaluated in comparison with clodronate. This therapy increased the median overall survival by 5.5 months. This study also noted the induction of a higher response rate in the cohort of elderly subjects who did not receive autologous transplantation in the zoledronic acid-treated group compared with the clodronate group.[13]

Zoledronic acid, therefore, has a significant role in the management of malignant bone disease and particularly remains a standard of care in the management of multiple myeloma patients.

DENOSUMAB

Denosumab is a RANKL inhibitor that is indicated for prevention of skeletal-related events in patients with bone metastases from solid tumors, treatment of adult and skeletally mature adolescents with giant cell tumor of bone that is unresectable, in cases in which surgical resection is likely to result in severe morbidity, and in treatment of hypercalcemia of malignancy refractory to bisphosphonate therapy.[14] Denosumab binds to RANKL, a transmembrane protein that is critical for the survival of osteoclasts. Denosumab prevents RANKL from activating receptor activator of nuclear factor κB (RANK), on the surface of osteoclasts and, therefore, modulates bone resorption and calcium release from the bone. It is administered using a subcutaneous route with a standard dose of 120 mg once every 4 weeks, when used for the management of malignant osteolytic bony disease.

Denosumab has been compared with zoledronic acid in multiple phase III trials evaluating subjects with metastatic breast cancer, metastatic castrate-resistant prostate cancer, and metastatic solid tumors including multiple myeloma.[15,16] Among all cohorts except multiple myeloma, denosumab was demonstrated to be either superior or noninferior to zoledronic acid. Mortality was noted to be higher with denosumab in a subgroup analysis of subjects with multiple myeloma and, therefore, at this time, its use is not recommended in patients with multiple myeloma outside of a clinical trial.

Denosumab has also been FDA approved at a lower dose of 60 mg subcutaneously every 6 months for the management of osteoporosis. In a double-blind multicenter study, denosumab administration was associated with increased bone mineral density and a reduction in the incidence of new vertebral fractures among men receiving androgen deprivation therapy for nonmetastatic prostate cancer.[17] However, the role of denosumab as a preventative agent for the development of metastatic disease has not yet been established. Similarly, in a randomized trial of denosumab in subjects receiving adjuvant aromatase inhibitors for nonmetastatic breast cancer, eligible women were assigned to receive placebo or subcutaneous denosumab 60 mg every 6 months. At 12 and 24 months, lumbar spine bone mineral density increased by 5.5% and 7.6%, respectively, in the denosumab group versus placebo. These studies demonstrate the ability of RANKL inhibitors to prevent and/or reverse the deleterious effect of antiandrogen antiestrogen therapies on bone health.[18]

Common adverse effects related to denosumab administration include hypocalcemia, hypersensitivity reactions, nausea, diarrhea, and musculoskeletal pain. Uncommon side effects include osteonecrosis of the jaw, atypical subtrochanteric and diaphyseal fracture, and hypersensitivity including anaphylactic reactions. In patients with severe renal dysfunction, the risk of hypocalcemia is noted to be higher. The pharmacokinetics of this agent are typically not affected with varying degrees of renal dysfunction. Due to the ease of its administration as a subcutaneous agent and its proven efficacy, it has become a treatment of choice for the management of metastatic bony disease for all solid tumors but not multiple myeloma, as previously discussed.

SUMMARY

Antiresorptive therapies such as bisphosphonates and RANKL inhibitor, denosumab, are an established standard of care in the management of malignant osteolytic bone disease. They have been shown to improve the quality of life of patients with cancer who have advanced bony disease and to attenuate the negative effects of antiandrogens on bone health in patients with prostate cancer and the effects of aromatase inhibitors in the management of breast cancer. In addition, bisphosphonates seems to have a role in improving survival in patients with multiple myeloma and may have a role in improving disease-free survival in the adjuvant therapy for hormone-sensitive breast cancer. It is, therefore, critically important to understand the cost-effectiveness and safety profile of these agents. Current laboratory investigations to understand their mechanism of action and clinical studies to optimize their indications, dosage schedule, and duration of therapy are ongoing. These will help elucidate their evolving role in the management of patients with malignant disease.

REFERENCES

1. Pamidronate Package Insert. March 2010. Available at: http://fresenius-kabi.ca/wp-content/uploads/2015/01/EN_Web_Insert_Pamid_NL.pdf.
2. Gucalp R, Ritch P, Wiernik PH, et al. Comparative study of pamidronate disodium and etidronate disodium in the treatment of cancer-related hypercalcemia. J Clin Oncol 1992;10(1):134–42.
3. Berenson JR, Lichtenstein A, Porter L, et al. Efficacy of pamidronate in reducing skeletal events in patients with advanced multiple myeloma. Myeloma Aredia Study Group. N Engl J Med 1996;334:488–93.
4. Hortobagyi GN, Theriault RL, Porter L, et al. Efficacy of pamidronate in reducing skeletal complications in patients with breast cancer and lytic bone metastases. Protocol 19 Aredia Breast Cancer Study Group. N Engl J Med 1996;335:1785–92.
5. Zoledronic Acid Package Insert. January 2015. Available at: https://www.pharma.us.novartis.com/product/pi/pdf/Zometa.pdf.
6. Major P, Lortholary A, Hon J, et al. Zoledronic acid is superior to pamidronate in the treatment of hypercalcemia of malignancy: a pooled analysis of two randomized, controlled clinical trials. J Clin Oncol 2001;19(2):558–67.
7. Gnant M, Mlineritsch B, Schippinger W, et al. Endocrine therapy plus zoledronic acid in premenopausal breast cancer. N Engl J Med 2009;360:679–91.

8. Coleman RE, Marshall H, Cameron D, et al. Breast-cancer adjuvant therapy with zoledronic acid. N Engl J Med 2011;365:1396–405.

9. Gralow J, Barlow WE, Paterson AH, et al. Phase III trial of bisphosphonates as adjuvant therapy in primary breast cancer: SWOG/Alliance/ECOG-ACRIN/NCIC Clinical trials group/NRG Oncology Study S0307. J Clin Oncol 2015;33 [suppl;abstr 503].

10. Smith MR, Halabi S, Ryan CJ, et al. Randomized controlled trial of early zoledronic acid in men with castration-sensitive prostate cancer and bone metastases: results of CALGB 90202 (Alliance). J Clin Oncol 2014;32(11):1143–50.

11. Rosen LS, Gordon D, Tchekmedyian S, et al. Zoledronic acid versus placebo in the treatment of skeletal metastases in patients with lung cancer and other solid tumors: a Phase III, double-blind, randomized trial—the Zoledronic Acid Lung Cancer and Other Solid Tumors Study Group. J Clin Oncol 2003;21(16):3150–7.

12. Himelstein LA, Qin R, Novotny PJ, et al. CALGB 70604 (Alliance): a randomized phase III study of standard dosing vs. longer interval dosing of zoledronic acid in metastatic cancer. J Clin Oncol 2015;33 [suppl; abstr 9501].

13. Morgan GJ, Davies FE, Gregory WM, et al. First-line treatment with zoledronic acid as compared with clodronic acid in multiple myeloma (MRC Myeloma IX): a randomised controlled trial. Lancet 2010;376: 1989–99.

14. Denosumab Package Insert. June 2015. Available at: http://pi.amgen.com/united_states/xgeva/xgeva_pi.pdf.

15. Stopeck AT, Lipton A, Body JJ, et al. Denosumab compared with zoledronic acid for the treatment of bone metastases in patients with advanced breast cancer: a randomized, double-blind study. J Clin Oncol 2010;28(35):5132–9.

16. Henry DH, Costa L, Goldwasser F, et al. Randomized, double-blind study of denosumab versus zoledronic acid in the treatment of bone metastases in patients with advanced cancer (excluding breast and prostate cancer) or multiple myeloma. J Clin Oncol 2011;29(9):1125–32.

17. Smith MR, Egerdie B, Toriz NH, et al. Denosumab in men receiving androgen-deprivation therapy for prostate cancer. N Engl J Med 2009;361:745–55.

18. Ellis GK, Bone HG, Chlebowski R, et al. Randomized trial of denosumab in patients receiving adjuvant aromatase inhibitors for nonmetastatic breast cancer. J Clin Oncol 2008;26(30):4875–82.

Indications and Outcomes of Osteoporosis and Bone Modulation Therapies

Stuart Weinerman, MD[a],*, Gianina L. Usera, MD[b]

KEYWORDS

- Bisphosphonates • Osteoporosis • Fracture • Bone mineral density • Anabolics • FRAX
- Glucocorticoids

KEY POINTS

- Osteoporosis-related fractures frequently go undiagnosed and untreated.
- There are many contributing factors of osteoporosis, including menopause, drugs, age, smoking, sedentary lifestyle, and sex, among others.
- Bone mineral density testing is a useful tool for health professionals to determine the need for treatment and also as a long-term monitoring tool.
- Calcium, vitamin D, and exercise, although popularly used as treatments for low bone density, have not been found to be effective in reducing the risk of fracture.

Osteoporosis is a skeletal disorder characterized by compromised bone strength predisposing to an increased risk of fracture.[1] This article addresses the causes of osteoporosis, how to identify who is at risk for fracture, and who should be considered for medical therapy for osteoporosis.

Osteoporosis-related fractures are a major public health issue, and are therefore an important topic for all health providers. For example, a 2004 report estimated 10 million Americans above age 50 have osteoporosis, leading to approximately 1.5 million fractures per year in the United States. Lifetime incidence of osteoporosis-related fractures is approximately 1 fracture per 2 women aged 50 years and older. Despite the public perception that this is a disease only a postmenopausal woman, the incidence in men is 1 fracture per 5 men. Osteoporosis-related fractures are associated with significant morbidity and mortality. Hip fractures in older women are associated with a 15% excess mortality; men with hip fractures have an even higher mortality, estimated at 30%.[2–4]

There are multiple causes of osteoporosis. The bone is a composite material of a collagen framework strengthened by hydroxyapatite, conceptually similar to concrete supported by a steel rebar. This composite material provides both resistance to deformity but still some flexibility. Bone biology depends on a balance of new bone formation, performed by osteoblasts, and resorption of old bone by osteoclasts, which allows growth and remodeling in response to stress or fracture repair. Osteocytes are osteoblasts that become embedded in the new bone. Rates of osteoclastic and osteoblastic activity are tightly linked in normal physiology. Bone remodeling begins with a signal to resorb an area of bone in

The authors report no financial or commercial conflicts of interest to disclose.
a Division of Endocrinology, Diabetes and Metabolism, Hofstra North Shore-LIJ School of Medicine, 865 Northern Boulevard, Suite 203, Great Neck, NY 11021, USA; b Division of Endocrinology, Diabetes and Metabolism, Department of Medicine, Hofstra North Shore-LIJ School of Medicine, 865 Northern Boulevard, Suite 203, Great Neck, NY 11021, USA
* Corresponding author.
E-mail address: sweinerm@nshs.edu

response to fracture or new stress. The osteo-blasts recruit new osteoclasts and stimulate resorption mainly through RANK-L (receptor activator for nuclear kappa beta ligand), under the influence of many of factors including sex hormones and parathyroid hormone. Osteoclasts, highly specialized cells, then resorb bone on the surface or tunneling through cortical bone. Osteoclasts form a tight seal on the bone, and then resorb the mineral with acid, and the protein matrix with proteases such as cathepsin K. The bone resorption phase lasts for approximately 3 weeks. Osteoblasts then migrate to the area and lay down new bone, first collagen matrix, which is then mineralized. Abnormalities of each phase and process of bone remodeling are represented by disease states, and are potential targets for pharmacologic therapy.

In childhood and adolescence, bone density increases as linear bone growth occurs. Peak bone density occurs slightly after linear growth stops, generally in the early 20s depending on the bone. Bone density tends to stay stable in healthy adults for several decades as long as there are normal sex steroid levels and circulation, estrogen in women and testosterone in men, and there are no other secondary risk factors such as inadequate nutrition or drugs that affect bone metabolism. Any cause of failure to achieve peak bone density will contribute to long-term risk of fractures (**Box 1**). Examples would include

---

Box 1
Risk factors for osteoporosis

- History of fracture
- Low bone mass
- Fracture in first-degree relative
- Female
- Low BMI
- Advanced age
- Menopause
- Cigarette smoking
- Excessive alcohol use
- Amenorrhea
- Anorexia nervosa
- Low lifetime calcium intake
- Vitamin D deficiency
- Certain drugs
- Low testosterone
- Sedentary lifestyle
- Caucasian or Asian

---

anorexia or chemotherapy in adolescence. Peak bone density appears to be genetically determined; approximately 60% of the variability between individuals appears to be familial. If peak bone density is normal, then the time or rate of bone loss later in life will contribute to the risk of fracture.

The most common cause of bone loss in otherwise healthy adults is the loss of estrogen at the time of menopause, whether a surgical or natural menopause. Any other cause of estrogen deficiency will also cause bone loss. This includes drug therapy such as aromatase inhibitors for breast cancer management, or Depo—Provera for contraception. The parallel is true in men. Low testosterone at any age is a contributor to bone loss.

There are numerous secondary causes for osteoporosis, some of which affect the bone quantity (ie, density), and some of which affect the bone quality, such as microarchitecture or bone mineral properties. Numerous disease states contribute to bone loss by a variety of mechanisms. These include a systemic inflammatory mechanism such as rheumatoid arthritis, secondary hypogonadism such as seen in Klinefelter syndrome or Turner syndrome, and nutritional abnormalities especially of calcium and vitamin D such as seen in celiac disease. Endocrinopathies can also contribute to osteoporosis. Examples include hyperparathyroidism with a direct increase in bone resorption, and Cushing syndrome with the effect of excess glucocorticoids on overall bone health, especially a decrease in osteoblastic function. Less common causes of osteoporosis include genetic abnormalities of the bone such as osteogenesis imperfecta, which is a defective synthesis of the bone collagen, or mastocytosis, a disease of rapid bone loss caused by localized release of inflammatory factors.

Numerous medications can also contribute to osteoporosis, through either a direct effect on bone or indirect effects through change in sex steroid levels or vitamin D levels. The most common is chronic use of glucocorticoids such as prednisone or hydrocortisone. Drugs that decrease sex hormone levels include aromatase inhibitors in breast cancer patients and androgen deprivation therapy in prostate cancer patients. Many other drugs also interfere with bone health (**Box 2**).

The major public health strategy is how to identify patients who are at risk for future fracture in order to target effective therapy and reduce risk. There have been multiple recommendations from a variety of international organizations on how to identify patients, yet osteoporosis remains inadequately diagnosed and treated, especially in high-risk patients.

Box 2
Medications that can contribute to osteoporosis

- Glucocorticoids
  - Prednisone
  - Hydrocortisone
- Aromatase Inhibitors
  - Arimidex
- Proton Pump Inhibitors
  - Pantoprazole
- Androgen Deprivation
  - Leuprolide
  - Goserelin
  - Triptorelin
  - Histrelin
  - Degarelix
  - Abiraterone
  - Flutamide
  - Bicalutamide
  - Nilutamide

The initial attempts to classify patients depended on bone density as the major identifiable risk factor. Dual energy x-ray absorptiometry is the standard test available for assessment of osteoporosis risk, as it is widely available, uses a very low dose radiograph, and can also be used to follow patients longitudinally.

Measurement of bone density is recommended for screening populations of patients at risk for fracture. The largest affected group is postmenopausal women. Screening is recommended for all women by age 65, earlier if other risk factors are also present, such as family history. In practice, many women are offered routine screening at menopause even if other risk factors are not present. Screening of premenopausal women without other risks, such as steroid use or anorexia, to determine the baseline, should be discouraged. Serial measurements allow monitoring the rate of bone loss over time. Repeat testing is often performed at 2 year intervals, but much longer intervals can be offered to low risk patients. Repeat testing at 1-year intervals is often used in high-risk situations such as use of glucocorticoids or to assess response to new medications.

Routine screening of healthy men remains controversial. There is good evidence that screening should begin at age 70 years in the absence of other risk factors, but third-party payers such as Medicare have not accepted this yet.[5,6] Many other populations should also be screened for osteoporosis. All patients with osteoporosis-related fractures, such vertebral or hip fractures in the elderly, should be considered as having osteoporosis and should be treated. Bone density testing can help guide therapy. Unfortunately most fracture patients do not get either bone density testing or medical therapy.

Special populations for testing include a wide variety of at-risk patients. All patients with sex hormone deficiency of any cause should be evaluated with bone densitometry, including, but not limited to patients with genetic disorders such as Turner or Klinefelter, anorexia nervosa, pituitary insufficiency, or drug-induced hypogonadism. Patients with disorders of calcium, parathyroid hormone, or vitamin D are at high risk for bone disease and should be screened. These disorders include celiac disease, hyperparathyroidism, short bowel syndrome, or gastric bypass surgery.

Good agreement exists concerning high-risk drugs. All patients, male or female, who are being treated with glucocorticoid therapy, at a dose of prednisone 5 mg/d or equivalent for 3 months or more, should be monitored with bone densitometry. All patients on aromatase inhibitor therapy or androgen deprivation should be evaluated. The threshold for treatment for these high-risk populations is different from the recommendations for more typical postmenopausal women, based on the higher risk of fracture. Glucocorticoid therapy, for example, induces early bone loss but also induces a qualitative abnormality. There is an increased risk of fracture even before bone density has decreased significantly.[7]

Many other drugs are associated with a lower risk of bone loss or fracture; there is little agreement concerning screening patients on these drugs. For example, proton pump inhibitors carry a small risk of bone loss, but this is not considered high enough to require bone density measurement in all patients on chronic therapy.

The World Health Organization (WHO) classifies postmenopausal osteoporosis as a T-score of less than 2.5 standard deviations. Based on a bone mineral density (BMD) scan, the T-score is a comparison of an individual's BMD with the mean value for young adults. Normal BMD is defined as greater than 1.0 standard deviation and above. Osteopenia, or low bone mass, falls into the category of being between -1.0 and -2.5 standard deviations of the mean of young adults.

The WHO classification was useful for standardization of diagnostic terms but is not adequate for predicting future fractures and selecting patients for therapy. The risk of fracture is increased not just with low bone density but numerous other factors. Predictors of future fracture include, in addition to low bone density, previous fractures, family history of fractures, especially hip fractures, increasing age, excessive alcohol use, and secondary risks caused by drug use or underlying diseases. These risks are synergistic, as shown in epidemiologic studies such as the Study of Osteoporotic Fractures. A model has been developed to help incorporate these risk factors into fracture prediction. The WHO has developed a model called FRAX, which can estimates the 10-year risk of a major fracture.[8] It can be helpful in situations when clinicians are unsure whether treatment for low bone density is warranted. Information needed to calculate the FRAX score are, age, sex, femoral neck bone density, body mass index (BMI), previous fragility fracture, family history of hip fracture, steroid use, smoking status, alcohol intake, rheumatoid arthritis, and whether there are any secondary causes of osteoporosis.

In 2008, the National Osteoporosis Foundation recommended initiating medical therapy for any patients at increased risk for fracture based on

1. Prior low trauma hip or vertebral fracture
2. Other prior fracture and low bone mass (T-score -1.0 to -2.5)
3. Osteoporosis by bone density criteria (ie, T-score less than −2.5)
4. Low bone mass and second-degree causes associated with high risk of fracture, such as other disease states or use of high-risk drugs
5. 10-year hip fracture probability of at least 3% or 10-year major osteoporosis-related fracture probability of at least 20%[9]

FRAX is only a guide, and does not cover a variety of scenarios, such as isolated low spine but normal hip BMD. Patches, or adjustments to FRAX, have been proposed but are not yet available.

Therapy for osteoporosis includes nutritional support, exercise, and medical therapy. Many patients rely on calcium, vitamin D, and other supplements for control of osteoporosis, despite a lack of evidence of benefits. The use of supplements has not been shown to be effective to prevent bone loss or reduce fractures in healthy, well-nourished patients. The Recommended Daily Allowance (RDA) for calcium is 1200 mg per day[10]; most women get 400 to 500 mg from diet, such as vegetables and grains. Dairy foods average 300 mg per serving, such as a glass of milk or container of yogurt. The authors generally recommend a supplement after estimating the patient's calcium intake; most women are offered 500 mg total

supplement (whether in a calcium tablet or multivitamin or both). More calcium has not been shown to improve bone health and may carry risk. The Women's Health Initiative (WHI) nutritional arm showed a small increase in kidney stone risk from calcium doses of 1000 mg compared with placebo.[11] A much larger controversy concerns whether calcium supplements increase cardiovascular risk, a question that has not yet been resolved.

Vitamin D also remains controversial. There is no doubt that adequate vitamin D is necessary for normal bone health, and that patients with low levels can develop secondary hyperparathyroidism or even rickets. The controversy relates to defining what is the normal range. The best measure of nutritional status of vitamin D is 25-hydroxy D, not the active 1,25 dihydroxy D, which is influenced by many hormonal factors. The Institute of Medicine (IOM) claimed that the lower limit of normal for 25-hydroxy D (25 Vit D) is 20 ng/mL[10]; other groups, such as the Endocrine Society claim 30 ng/mL as a more reasonable threshold.[12] The need for vitamin D supplementation will differ greatly depending on the levels targeted. This debate will only be resolved when prospective randomized outcome studies are completed. The authors generally recommend 1000 IU per day of vitamin D as a supplement. There are inadequate data to prefer vitamin D2, ergocalciferol (from plant sources) versus vitamin D3, cholecalciferol (from animal sources), although many claims for vitamin D3 have been made. Many other supplements are available in health food stores and are added to a variety of bone support preparations. These include boron, vitamin K, manganese, and strontium. There is no evidence to support the use of these supplements.

Exercise is an important component of a plan to reduce fractures. The effect on bone density is less than most people hope, but it may reduce fractures by reducing muscular frailty, improving balance, and reducing falls. Unfortunately, the combination of calcium, vitamin D, and exercise will not be adequate to prevent bone loss and reduce fractures for most patients with osteoporosis, despite what is written in the lay press. Medical therapy will be required for most patients at increased risk. Fortunately, there are now multiple options for treatment on the horizon, with newer drugs targeting different mechanisms.

The 2 main types of therapy currently available for osteoporosis can be divided into antiresorptive medications and anabolic agents. Antiresorptive drugs target the osteoclasts and directly reduce bone resorption; these include estrogens, selective estrogen-receptor modulators (SERMS), bisphosphonatoo, denosumab, and calcitonin. Osteoblastic bone formation is tightly linked to resorptive activity; suppression of resorption is highly linked to suppression of formation, which may be a critical factor in the development of adverse effects of long-term potent antiresorptives such as bisphosphonates, namely osteonecrosis of the jaw (ONJ) and atypical femur fractures (further information is available in the article on antiresorptive therapy by Dr. Weinerman and Dr. Usera elsewhere in this issue). The only US Food and Drug Administration (FDA)-approved directly anabolic agent is teriparatide, the 1 to 34 amino acid fragment of parathyroid hormone.

The most promising newer pharmacologic agents include cathepsin K inhibitors and anti-sclerostin antibodies. Cathepsin K is a protease secreted by the osteoclasts into the bone resorptive space responsible for removing the protein matrix in bone; hydrogen ions secreted by the osteoclasts resorb the mineral component. Odanacatib inhibits this enzyme, reducing bone resorption without turning off the osteoclast, which allows persistent normal osteoblast activity; this is the first drug to allow uncoupling of the bone remodeling cycle. A large phase 3 trial showed good increase in bone density and reductions of fractures, but has not yet been submitted to the FDA for approval (as of this writing, March 2015).[13]

Antisclerostin antibody therapy targets a process within the WNT signaling process, which is crucial for modulation of bone remodeling. Preliminary data with 2 agents suggest marked increases in bone formation and increases in bone density, with potency not available with current therapies.

In summary, fractures caused by osteoporosis are common and represent a public health risk that should be of concern to all health professionals. Identification of patients at risk for fractures can be made based on clinical risk factors as well as bone density testing. Testing and treatment are underutilized in the groups at highest risk, such as hip fracture patients. Many patients hope or expect that calcium, vitamin D, and exercise will be adequate to treat osteoporosis, but the evidence does not support this. Excellent treatment options that have been clearly shown to reduce fractures are available, but are not popular with patients due to fears of long-term complications. Newer therapies may offer more potent or possibly safer options.

REFERENCES

1. Osteoporosis prevention, diagnosis, and therapy. NIH Consens Statement 2000;17(1):1–36.
2. Cawthon PM, Ensrud KE, Laughlin GA, et al. Sex hormones and frailty in older men: the osteoporotic fractures in men (MrOS) study. J Clin Endocrinol Metab 2009;94(10):3806–15.
3. Mellstrom D, Johnell O, Ljunggren O, et al. Free testosterone is an independent predictor of BMD and prevalent fractures in elderly men: MrOs Sweden. J Bone Miner Res 2006;21(4):529–35.
4. Seeman E, Delmas PD. Bone quality- the material and structural basis of bone strength and fragility. N Engl J Med 2006;354(21):2250–61.
5. Kenny AM, Gallagher JC, Prestwood KM, et al. Bone density, bone turnover, and hormone levels in men over 75. J Gerontol A Biol Sci Med Sci 1998;53(6):M419–25.
6. Watts NB, Adler RA, Bilezikian JP, et al. Osteoporosis in men: an Endocrine Society clinical practice guideline. J Clin Endocrinol Metab 2012;97(6):1802–22.
7. Grossman JM, Gordon R, Ranganath VK, et al. ACR 2010 recommendations for prevention and treatment of glucocorticoid-induced osteoporosis. Arthritis Care Res 2010;62(11):1515–26.
8. Siris ES, Baim S, Nattiv A. Primary care use of FRAX: absolute fracture risk assessment in postmenopausal women and older men. Postgrad Med 2010;122(1):82–90.
9. National Osteoporosis Foundation. Clinician's guide to prevention and treatment of osteoporosis. Washington, DC: National Osteoporosis Foundation; 2010.
10. Ross AC, Taylor CL, Yaktine AL, et al, editors. Committee to review dietary reference intakes for Vitamin D and Calcium. IOM; 2010.
11. Heaney RP. Calcium supplementation and incident kidney stone risk: a systematic review. J Am Coll Nutr 2008;27(5):519–27.
12. Holick MF, Binkley MC. Evaluation, treatment and prevention of vitamin D deficiency: an Endocrine Society Clinical Practice Guideline. J Clin Endocrinol Metab 2011;96(7):1911–30.
13. Zerbini CA, McClung MR. Odanacatib in postmenopausal women with low bone mineral density: a review of current clinical evidence. Ther Adv Musculoskelet Dis 2013;5(4):199–209.

Index

Note: Page numbers of article titles are in **boldface** type.

oralmaxsurgery.theclinics.com

United States Postal Service

Statement of Ownership, Management, and Circulation
(All Periodicals Publications Except Requestor Publications)

1. Publication Title	2. Publication Number								3. Filing Date
Oral and Maxillofacial Surgery Clinics of North America	0	0	6	-	3	6	2		9/18/15

4. Issue Frequency	5. Number of Issues Published Annually	6. Annual Subscription Price
Feb, May, Aug, Nov	4	$385.00

7. Complete Mailing Address of Known Office of Publication (Not printer) (Street, city, county, state, and ZIP+4®)

Elsevier Inc.
360 Park Avenue South
New York, NY 10010-1710

Contact Person
Stephen R. Bushing

Telephone (Include area code)
215-239-3688

8. Complete Mailing Address of Headquarters or General Business Office of Publisher (Not printer)

Elsevier Inc., 360 Park Avenue South, New York, NY 10010-1710

9. Full Names and Complete Mailing Addresses of Publisher, Editor, and Managing Editor (Do not leave blank)

Publisher (Name and complete mailing address)

Linda Belfus, Elsevier Inc., 1600 John F. Kennedy Blvd., Ste. 1800, Philadelphia, PA 19103-2899

Editor (Name and complete mailing address)

John Vassallo, Elsevier Inc., 1600 John F. Kennedy Blvd., Ste. 1800, Philadelphia, PA 19103-2899

Managing Editor (Name and complete mailing address)

Adrienne Brigido, Elsevier Inc., 1600 John F. Kennedy Blvd., Ste. 1800, Philadelphia, PA 19103-2899

10. Owner (Do not leave blank. If the publication is owned by a corporation, give the name and address of the corporation immediately followed by the names and addresses of all stockholders owning or holding 1 percent or more of the total amount of stock. If not owned by a corporation, give the names and addresses of the individual owners. If owned by a partnership or other unincorporated firm, give its name and address as well as those of each individual owner. If the publication is published by a nonprofit organization, give its name and address.)

Full Name	Complete Mailing Address
Wholly owned subsidiary of	1600 John F. Kennedy Blvd, Ste. 1800
Reed/Elsevier, US holdings	Philadelphia, PA 19103-2899

11. Known Bondholders, Mortgagees, and Other Security Holders Owning or Holding 1 Percent or More of Total Amount of Bonds, Mortgages, or Other Securities. If none, check box ☐ None

Full Name	Complete Mailing Address
N/A	

12. Tax Status (For completion by nonprofit organizations authorized to mail at nonprofit rates) (Check one)
The purpose, function, and nonprofit status of this organization and the exempt status for federal income tax purposes:
☐ Has Not Changed During Preceding 12 Months
☐ Has Changed During Preceding 12 Months (Publisher must submit explanation of change with this statement)

PS Form 3526, July 2014 (Page 1 of 3 (Instructions Page 3)) PSN 7530-01-000-9931 PRIVACY NOTICE: See our Privacy policy in www.usps.com

---

13. Publication Title	14. Issue Date for Circulation Data Below
Oral and Maxillofacial Surgery Clinics of North America	August 2015

15. Extent and Nature of Circulation			Average No. Copies Each Issue During Preceding 12 Months	No. Copies of Single Issue Published Nearest to Filing Date
a. Total Number of Copies (Net press run)			1342	1203
b. Legitimate Paid and Or Requested Distribution (By Mail and Outside the Mail)	(1)	Mailed Outside-County Paid/Requested Mail Subscriptions stated on PS Form 3541. (Include paid distribution above nominal rate, advertiser's proof copies and exchange copies)	919	819
	(2)	Mailed In-County Paid/Requested Mail Subscriptions stated on PS Form 3541. (Include paid distribution above nominal rate, advertiser's proof copies and exchange copies)		
	(3)	Paid Distribution Outside the Mails Including Sales Through Dealers And Carriers, Street Vendors, Counter Sales, and Other Paid Distribution Outside USPS®	170	193
	(4)	Paid Distribution by Other Classes of Mail Through the USPS (e.g. First-Class Mail®)		
c. Total Paid and or Requested Circulation (Sum of 15b (1), (2), (3), and (4))		↑	1089	1012
d. Free or Nominal Rate Distribution (By Mail and Outside the Mail)	(1)	Free or Nominal Rate Outside-County Copies included on PS Form 3541	62	57
	(2)	Free or Nominal Rate In-County Copies included on PS Form 3541		
	(3)	Free or Nominal Rate Copies mailed at Other classes Through the USPS (e.g. First-Class Mail®)		
	(4)	Free or Nominal Rate Distribution Outside the Mail (Carriers or Other means)		
e. Total Nonrequested Distribution (Sum of 15d (1), (2), (3) and (4))			62	57
f. Total Distribution (Sum of 15c and 15e)		↑	1151	1069
g. Copies not Distributed (See instructions to publishers #4 (page #3))		↑	191	134
h. Total (Sum of 15f and g)		↑	1342	1203
i. Percent Paid and/or Requested Circulation (15c divided by 15f times 100)		↑	94.61%	94.67%

* If you are claiming electronic copies go to line 16 on page 3. If you are not claiming Electronic copies, skip to line 17 on page 3.

16. Electronic Copy Circulation	Average No. Copies Each Issue During Preceding 12 Months	No. Copies of Single Issue Published Nearest to Filing Date
a. Paid Electronic Copies		
b. Total paid Print Copies (Line 15c) + Paid Electronic copies (Line 16a)		
c. Total Print Distribution (Line 15f) + Paid Electronic Copies (Line 16a)		
d. Percent Paid (Both Print & Electronic copies) (16b divided by 16c X 100)		

☐ I certify that 50% of all my distributed copies (electronic and print) are paid above a nominal price

17. Publication of Statement of Ownership
If the publication is a general publication, publication of this statement is required. Will be printed in the _November 2015_ issue of this publication.

18. Signature and Title of Editor, Publisher, Business Manager, or Owner	Date
Stephen R. Bushing	September 18, 2015
Stephen R. Bushing – Inventory Distribution Coordinator	

I certify that all information furnished on this form is true and complete. I understand that anyone who furnishes false or misleading information on this form or who omits material or information requested on the form may be subject to criminal sanctions (including fines and imprisonment) and/or civil sanctions (including civil penalties).

PS Form 3526, July 2014 (Page 3 of 3)

Moving?

Make sure your subscription moves with you!

To notify us of your new address, find your **Clinics Account Number** (located on your mailing label above your name), and contact customer service at:

Email: journalscustomerservice-usa@elsevier.com

800-654-2452 (subscribers in the U.S. & Canada)
314-447-8871 (subscribers outside of the U.S. & Canada)

Fax number: 314-447-8029

Elsevier Health Sciences Division
Subscription Customer Service
3251 Riverport Lane
Maryland Heights, MO 63043

*To ensure uninterrupted delivery of your subscription,
please notify us at least 4 weeks in advance of move.

Printed and bound by CPI Group (UK) Ltd, Croydon, CR0 4YY

03/10/2024

01040375-0007